AACN Pocket Handbook of
Critical Care Nursing

AACN Pocket Handbook of
Critical Care Nursing

Marianne Chulay, RN, DNSc, FAAN
Consultant, Critical Care Nursing and Clinical Research, Chapel Hill, North Carolina
Director, Nursing Research and Practice
Moses Cone Health System
Greensboro, North Carolina

Cathie Guzzetta, RN, PhD, FAAN
Director, Holistic Nursing Consultants
Nursing Research Consultant
Parkland Memorial Hospital and Children's Medical Center
Dallas, Texas

Barbara Dossey, RN, MS, FAAN
Director, Holistic Nursing Consultants
Santa Fe, New Mexico
Co-Director, BodyMind Systems
Temple, Texas

APPLETON & LANGE
Stamford, CT

Notice: The authors and the publisher of this volume have taken care to make certain that the doses of drugs and schedules of treatment are correct and compatible with the standards generally accepted at the time of publication. Nevertheless, as new information becomes available, changes in treatment and in the use of drugs become necessary. The reader is advised to carefully consult the instruction and information material included in the package insert of each drug or therapeutic agent before administration. This advice is especially important when using, administering, or recommending new or infrequently used drugs. The authors and publisher disclaim all responsibility for any liability, loss, injury, or damage incurred as a consequence, directly or indirectly, of the use and application of any of the contents of this volume.

Prentice Hall International (UK) Limited, *London*
Prentice Hall of Australia Pty. Limited, *Sydney*
Prentice Hall Canada, Inc., *Toronto*
Prentice Hall Hispanoamericana, S.A., *Mexico*
Prentice Hall of India Private Limited, *New Delhi*
Prentice Hall of Japan, Inc., *Tokyo*
Simon & Schuster Asia Pte. Ltd., *Singapore*
Editora Prentice Hall do Brasil Ltda., *Rio de Janiero*
Prentice Hall, *Upper Saddle River, New Jersey*

ISBN 0-8385-0322-5

Library of Congress Catalog Card Number:
97-071823

Editor: David P. Carroll
Production: Andover Publishing Services
Designer: Janice Barsevich Bielawa
Original Illustrations: Kerry Bassett, Raleigh, NC

PRINTED IN THE UNITED STATES OF AMERICA

To our critical care nursing colleagues around the world
who journey on the path of caring, healing, and excellence.

Contents

Contributors

Michael H. Ackerman, DNS, RN, CCRN
Advanced Practice Nurse/Critical Care
Strong Memorial Hospital
Associate Professor of Clinical Nursing
School of Nursing
University of Rochester
Rochester, New York

Thomas Ahrens, RN, DNSc
Clinical Nurse Specialist, MICU
Barnes Hospital
St. Louis, Missouri

Sandi O'Brien Brettler, RN, MSN, CCRN
Clinical Nurse Specialist, Neuroscience
Moses Cone Health System
Greensboro, North Carolina

Suzanne M. Burns, RN, MSN, RRT, CCRN, ACNP
Clinician 5 and Associate Professor of Nursing
School of Nursing
University of Virginia Health Sciences Center
Charlottesville, Virginia

Debra Byram, RN, MS
Clinical Nurse Specialist
Warren G. Magnuson Clinical Center
National Institutes of Health
Bethesda, Maryland

Karen K. Carlson, RN, MN
Critical Care Clinical Nurse Specialist
The Carlson Consultant Group
Bellevue, Washington and
Clinical Faculty, School of Nursing
University of Washington
Seattle, Washington

Marianne Chulay, RN, DNSc, FAAN
Consultant, Critical Care Nursing and
 Clinical Research
Chapel Hill, North Carolina
and
Director, Nursing Research and Practice
Moses Cone Health System
Greensboro, North Carolina

Maria A. Connolly, RN, DNSc, CCRN
Associate Professor of Medical-Surgical
 Nursing
Niehoff School of Nursing
Loyola University of Chicago
Chicago, Illinois

Barbara Dossey, RN, MS, FAAN
Director, Holistic Nursing Consultants
Santa Fe, New Mexico
Co-Director, BodyMind Systems
Temple, Texas

Dorrie K. Fontaine, RN, DNSc, FAAN
Clinical Associate Professor
Coordinator, Acute Care Nurse Practitioner
 Program
School of Nursing
Georgetown University
Washington, DC

Bradi Bartrug Granger, RN, MSN
Clinical Nurse Specialist, Cardiology
Duke University Medical Center
Durham, North Carolina

**Ann Smith Gregoire, RN, MSN, CRNP,
 CCRN**
Clinical Nurse Specialist
Surgical Intensive Care Unit
Thomas Jefferson University Hospital
Philadelphia, Pennsylvania

Cathie Guzzetta, RN, PhD, FAAN
Director, Holistic Nursing Consultants
Nursing Research Consultant
Parkland Memorial Hospital and Children's
 Medical Center
Dallas, Texas

Carol Jacobson, RN, MN, CCRN
Director, Quality Educational Services
Critical Care Consultant and Educator
Seattle, Washington

Susan Johnson, RN, MSN
Unit Manager, Infectious Disease Unit
University of Syracuse Hospital System
Syracuse, New York

Deborah G. Klein, RN, MSN, CCRN, CS
Clinical Nurse Specialist
Trauma/Critical Care Nursing
MetroHealth Medical Center
Cleveland, Ohio

Joanne Krumberger, RN, MS, CCRN
Critical Care Clinical Nurse Specialist
Clement J. Zablocky Veterans Affairs
  Medical Center
Milwaukee, Wisconsin

Debra J. Lynn-McHale, RN, MSN, CS, CCRN
Staff Development Coordinator
Thomas Jefferson University Hospital
Philadelphia, Pennsylvania

Diane J. Mick, MSN, RN, CCRN
Doctoral Student
Research Assistant
School of Nursing
University of Rochester
Rochester, New York

Mary Beth Egloff Parr, MSN, RN, CCRN
Senior Clinical Nurse Specialist and
  Educator
Pulmonary and Special Services
Sharp Health Care
San Diego, California

Carol A. Rauen, RN, MS, CCRN
Nursing Coordinator and Clinical Nurse
  Specialist
Georgetown University Hospital
Washington, DC

Juanita Reigle, RN, MSN, CCRN, ACNP
Clinician 5, Cardiology
Assistant Professor of Nursing
School of Nursing
University of Virginia Health Sciences
  Center
Charlottesville, Virginia

Anita Sherer, RN, MSN
Clinical Pathway Coordinator
Moses Cone Health System
Greensboro, North Carolina

Sue Simmons-Alling, RN, MSN
Advanced Practice Psychiatric Nurse
Therapist
Spring Lake Heights, New Jersey

Gerrye Stegall, RN, MN, CCRN
Research Coordinator
East Alabama Medical Center
Opelika, Alabama

Gregory M. Susla, PharmD, FCCM
Critical Care Pharmacist
Warren G. Magnuson Clinical Center
National Institutes of Health
Bethesda, Maryland

Debbie Tribett, MS, RN, CS, LNP
Adult Nurse Practitioner
Infectious Diseases Physicians
Fairfax, Virginia

Lorie Rietman Wild, RN, MN
Clinical Nurse Specialist
University of Washington Medical Center
Seattle, Washington

Susan L. Woods, PhD, RN
Professor of Nursing
Department of Biobehavioral Nursing and
    Health Systems
School of Nursing
University of Washington
Seattle, Washington

Marlene S. Yates, RN, BSN
Clinical Nurse Educator
Moses Cone Health System
Greensboro, North Carolina

Preface

Given the complexity of critical care practice today, it's impossible for even experienced clinicians to remember all the information required to give safe and effective care to critically ill patients. Clinicians frequently need to use a variety of clinical resources to verify drug information, normal laboratory and physiologic values, ECG and hemodynamic monitoring information, emergency algorithms, and other essential facts of patient management.

To save time and avoid frustration, clinicians often create their own "pocket guides" by cutting and pasting together information from a variety of sources so they always have a quick reference source available. The *AACN Pocket Handbook of Critical Care Nursing* is designed to provide busy clinicians with an easy to use resource that can, literally, be kept in their pockets. The pocket handbook contains selected tables and figures from the textbook, *AACN Hand-book of Critical Care Nursing* (Appleton & Lange, Stamford, CT, 1997), and includes items that clinicians are most likely to need at their fingertips:

- Critical care drug tables (common vasoactive drugs, neuromuscular blocking agents, antiarrhythmics, IV medication guidelines)
- Normal values table for laboratory tests and physiologic parameters
- Lists of assessment components

- Cardiac rhythms: ECG characteristics and treatment guides including sample rhythm strips
- 12-lead ECG changes in acute myocardial ischemia and infarct
- Troubleshooting guides for ventilators and hemodynamic monitoring equipment
- Guide to alternative complementary therapies (imagery, relaxation, music therapy, touch)

- Indications for mechanical ventilation
- Weaning assessment tool
- Chest x-ray interpretation
- Managing enteral feeding complications
- Guidelines for the transfer of critically ill patients
- Blank pages for you to write in important phone numbers and add other information to individualize your pocket guide

We hope this pocket book will, indeed, be placed in your pocket and assist you in making a difference in the lives of the patients and families you encounter.

Marianne Chulay
Cathie Guzzetta
Barbara Dossey

Normal Values

1.1 ▶ Normal Values Table

Abbreviation	Definition	Normal Value
BSA	Body surface area (Value obtained from a nomogram based on height and weight)	Meters squared (m^2)
MAP	Mean systemic arterial pressure (MAP estimate = diastolic pressure + 1/3 pulse pressure)	85–90 mm Hg
CVP	Central venous pressure	5–12 cm H_2O
PA	Mean pulmonary artery pressure	10–17 mm Hg
PCWP	Mean pulmonary capillary wedge pressure	5–12 mm Hg
CO	Cardiac output	5–6 L/minute
CI	Cardiac index $$CI \ (L/minute/m^2) = \frac{cardiac\ output\ (L/minute)}{body\ surface\ area\ (m^2)}$$	2.5–3.5 L/minute/m^2
SVR	Systemic vascular resistance $$SVR \ (TPR) \ (dynes/second/cm^5) = \frac{(MAP \ [mm \ Hg] - CVP \ [mm \ Hg]) \times 79.9}{cardiac\ output\ (L/minute)}$$	900–1200 dynes/second/cm^5
PVR	Pulmonary vascular resistance $$PVR \ (dynes/second/cm^5) = \frac{(PA \ [mm \ Hg] - PCWP \ [mm \ Hg]) \times 79.9}{cardiac\ output\ (L/minute)}$$	120–200 dynes/second/cm^5
HR	Heart rate	60–90 beats/minute

Adapted from: Hall J, Schmidt G, Wood L. Principles of critical care. New York: McGraw Hill, 1993, cover tables I–IV.

Abbreviation	Definition	Normal Value
SV	Stroke volume $$SV\ (ml/beat) = \frac{cardiac\ output\ (ml)}{heart\ rate}$$	50–100 ml/beat
SI	Stroke index $$SI\ (ml/minute/m^2) = \frac{stroke\ volume}{body\ surface\ area}$$	35–50 ml/m^2
RVSW	Right ventricular stroke work $RVSW = SI \times MPAP \times 0.0144$	51–61 g/m/m^2
LVSW	Left ventricular stroke work $LVSW = SI \times MAP \times 0.0144$	8–10 g/m/m^2
EF	Ejection fraction $$Ejection\ fraction = \frac{SV}{EDV}$$	70%
EDV	End-diastolic volume	50–90 ml
dp/dt	First time derivative of left ventricular pressure	13–14 seconds
P$_{AO_2}$	Mean partial pressure of oxygen in alveolus	104 mm Hg
P$_{ACO_2}$	Partial pressure of carbon dioxide in alveolus	40 mm Hg
Pao$_2$	Partial pressure of oxygen in arterial blood	Will vary with patient's age and the FiO$_2$. On room air: 80–95 mm Hg. On 100% O$_2$: 640 mm Hg.
Paco$_2$	Partial pressure of carbon dioxide in arterial blood	35–45 mm Hg

1.1 ► Normal Values Table *(continued)*

Abbreviation	Definition	Normal Value
Pvo_2	Partial pressure of oxygen in mixed venous blood	Will vary with the FiO_2, cardiac output, and oxygen consumption from 35–40 mm Hg
$Pvco_2$	Partial pressure of carbon dioxide in mixed venous blood	41–51 mm Hg
$P(A-a)o_2$	Alveolar-arterial oxygen gradient $P(A-a)o_2$ (mm Hg) = $PAo_2 - Pao_2$	25–65 mm Hg at $FiO_2 = 1.0$
Sao_2	Percentage of oxyhemoglobin saturation of arterial blood	97% (air)
Svo_2	Percentage of oxyhemoglobin saturation of mixed venous blood	75% (air)
Cao_2	Arterial oxygen content	Will vary with hemoglobin concentration and Pao_2 on air from 19–20 ml/100 ml
	Cao_2 (ml O_2/100 ml blood or vol %) = (Hb × 1.39) SaO_2 + (Pao_2 × 0.0031)	
Cvo_2	Mixed venous oxygen content	Will vary with Cao_2, cardiac output, and O_2 consumption from 14–15 ml/100 ml
$C(a-v)o_2$	Arteriovenous oxygen content difference $C(a-v)o_2$ (ml/100 ml or vol %) = $Cao_2 - Cvo_2$	4–6 ml/100 ml
O_2 avail	Oxygen availability O_2 avail (ml/minute/m^2) = CI × Cao_2 × 10	550–650 ml/minute/m^2
O_2 ext ratio	Oxygen extraction ratio O_2 ext ratio = $\dfrac{C(a-v)o_2}{Cao_2}$	0.25
P_B	Barometric pressure	

Abbreviation	Definition	Normal Value
V_{O_2}	Oxygen consumption	115–165 ml/minute/m^2
	O_2 ext ratio $= \dfrac{C(a-v)_{O_2}}{Ca_{O_2}}$	
V_{CO_2}	Carbon dioxide production	192 ml/minute
R or RQ	Respiratory quotient	0.8
	$RQ = \dfrac{V_{CO_2}}{V_{O_2}}$	
FRC	Functional residual capacity	2400 ml
VC	Vital capacity	65–75 ml/kg
IF	Inspiratory force	75–100 cm H_2O
EDC	Effective dynamic compliance	35–45 ml/cm H_2O females 40–50 ml/cm H_2O males
	$EDC \ (ml/cm \ H_2O) = \dfrac{tidal \ volume \ (ml)}{peak \ airway \ pressure \ (cm \ H_2O)}$	
V_D	Dead space	150 ml
	$Vd/Vt = \dfrac{Pa_{CO_2} - Pe_{CO_2}}{Pa_{CO_2}}$	
V_T	Tidal volume	500 ml

1.1 ► Normal Values Table *(continued)*

Abbreviation	Definition	Normal Value
V_D/V_T	Dead space to tidal volume ratio	0.25–0.40
Q_S/Q_T	Right-to-left shunt (percentage of cardiac output flowing past nonventilated alveoli or the equivalent) $$Q_S/Q_T(\%) = \frac{0.0031 \times P(A-a)o_2}{C(a-v)O_2 + (0.0031 \times P[A-a]o_2)} \times 100$$ Valid only when arterial blood is 100% saturated	5–8%

Assessment

2.1 ▶ Prearrival and Admission Quick Check Assessments

Prearrival Assessment
- Abbreviated report on patient (age, sex, chief complaint, diagnosis, pertinent history, physiologic status, invasive devices, equipment, and status of laboratory/diagnostic tests
- Room setup complete, including verification of proper equipment functioning

Admission Quick Check Assessment
- General appearance (consciousness)
- *A*irway:
  Patency
  Position of artificial airway (if present)
- *B*reathing:
  Quantity and quality of respirations (rate, depth, pattern, symmetry, effort, use of accessory muscles)
  Breath sounds
  Presence of spontaneous breathing
- *C*irculation and *C*erebral Perfusion:
  ECG (rate, rhythm, and presence of ectopy)
  Blood pressure
  Peripheral pulses and capillary refill
  Presence of bleeding
  Level of consciousness, responsiveness
- *C*hief Complaint:
  Primary body system
  Associated symptoms

- *D*rugs and *D*iagnostic Tests:
  Drugs prior to admission (prescribed, over-the-counter, illegal)
  Current medications
  Review diagnostic test results
- *E*quipment:
  Patency of vascular and drainage systems
  Appropriate functioning and labeling of all equipment connected to patient
- Allergies

2.2 ► Comprehensive Admission Assessment

Past Medical History
Medical conditions, surgical procedures
Psychiatric/emotional problems
Hospitalizations
Previous medications (prescription, over-the-counter, illicit drugs) and time of last medication dose
Allergies
Review of body systems (see Section 2.3)

Social History
Age, sex
Ethnic origin
Height, weight
Highest educational level completed
Occupation
Marital status
Primary family members/significant others
Religious affiliation
Durable power of attorney (DPA) or living will
Substance use (alcohol, drugs, caffeine, tobacco)

Family History
Cancer, heart disease, hypertension, diabetes, seizures, stroke, or ulcers

Psychosocial Assessment
Mental status
General communication
Coping styles
Perception of illness
Expectations of critical care unit
Current stresses
Family needs

Spirituality
Meaning and purpose
Inner strength
Inner connections

Physical Assessment
Nervous system
Cardiovascular system
Respiratory system
Renal system
Gastrointestinal system
Endocrine, hematologic, and immune systems
Integumentary system

2.3 ► Review of Past History

Body System	History Questions
Nervous	• Have you ever had a seizure? • Have you ever fainted, blacked out, or had delirium tremens (DTs)? • Do you ever have numbness, tingling, or weakness in any part of your body? • Do you have any difficulty with your hearing, vision, or speech? • Has your daily activity level changed due to your present condition? • Do you require any assistive devices such as canes?
Cardiovascular	• Have you experienced any heart problems or disease such as heart attacks? • Do you have any problems with extreme fatigue? • Do you have an irregular heart rhythm? • Do you have high blood pressure? • Do you have a pacemaker or an implanted defibrillator?
Respiratory	• Do you ever experience shortness of breath? • Do you have any pain associated with breathing? • Do you have a persistent cough? Is it productive? • Have you had any exposure to environmental agents that might affect the lungs?
Renal	• Have you had any change in frequency of urination? • Do you have any burning, pain, discharge, or difficulty when you urinate? • Have you had blood in your urine?

Body System	History Questions
Gastrointestinal	• Has there been any recent weight loss or gain? • Have you had any change in appetite? • Do you have any problems with nausea or vomiting? • How often do you have a bowel movement and has there been a change in the normal pattern? Do you have blood in your stools? • Do you have dentures?
Integumentary	• Do you have any problems with your skin?
Endocrine and Hematologic	• Do you have any problems with bleeding?
Immunologic	• Do you have problems with chronic infections?

2.3 ▸ Review of Past History *(continued)*

Body System	History Questions
Psychosocial	• Do you have any physical conditions which make communication difficult (hearing loss, visual disturbances, language barriers, etc.)?
	• Is it difficult for you to ask questions or let others know what you need?
	• How do you best learn? Do you need information repeated several times and/or require information in advance of teaching sessions?
	• What are the ways you cope with stress, crises, or pain?
	• Who are the important people in your "family" or network? Who do you want to make decisions with you, or for you?
	• Have you had any previous experiences with critical illness?
	• Have you ever been abused?
	• Do you have problems with attention, problem solving, or memory?
	• Have you ever experienced trouble with agitation, irritability, being confused, mood swings, or suicide attempts?
	• What is the impact of illness on the family?
	• What are the cultural practices, religious influences, and values that are important to the family?
	• What are family members' perceptions and expectations of the critical care staff and the setting?
	• What are the crisis or coping skills of family members?
	• What are the learning styles of family members?

Body System	History Questions
Spiritual*	Meaning and purpose: • What gives your life meaning? • Do you have a sense of purpose in life? • Does your illness interfere with your life goals? • Why do you want to get well? • How hopeful are you about obtaining a better degree of health? • What is the most motivating or powerful thing in your life? Inner strengths: • What brings you joy and peace in your life? • What are your personal strengths? • What do you believe in? • Is faith important to you? • How has your illness influenced your faith? • Does faith play a role in regaining your health? Interconnections: • How do you feel about yourself right now? • What do you do to heal your spirit?

*Adapted from: Guzzetta C, Dossey B: Cardiovascular nursing: Holistic practice. *St. Louis, MO: Mosby-Year Book, 1992, p. 9.*

2.4 ▶ Ongoing Assessment Template

Body System	Assessment Parameters
Nervous	• LOC • Pupils • Motor strength of extremities
Cardiovascular	• Blood pressure • Heart rate and rhythm • Heart sounds • Capillary refill • Peripheral pulses • Patency of IVs • Verification of IV solutions and medications • Hemodynamic pressures and waveforms • Cardiac output data
Respiratory	• Respiratory rate and rhythm • Breath sounds • Color and amount of secretions • Noninvasive technology information (e.g., pulse oximetry, end-tidal CO_2) • Mechanical ventilatory parameters • Arterial and venous blood gases
Renal	• Intake and output • Color and amount of urinary output • BUN/creatinine values

2.4 ► Ongoing Assessment Template (continued)

Body System	Assessment Parameters
Gastrointestinal	• Bowel sounds • Contour of abdomen • Position of drainage tubs • Color and amount of secretions • Bilirubin and albumin values
Endocrine, Hematologic, and Immunologic	• Fluid balance • Electrolyte and glucose values • CBC and coagulation values • Temperature • WBC with differential count
Integumentary	• Color and temperature of skin • Intactness of skin • Areas of redness
Pain/discomfort	• Assessed in each system
Psychosocial	• Mental status and behavioral responses • Reaction to critical illness experience (e.g., stress, anxiety, coping, mood) • Presence of cognitive impairments (dementia, delirium), depression, or demoralization • Family functioning and needs • Ability to communicate needs and participate in care • Sleep patterns

2.5 ► Symptom Assessment

Characteristic	Sample Questions
Onset	How and under what circumstances did it begin? Was the onset sudden or gradual? Did it progress?
Location	Where is it? Does it stay in the same place or does it radiate or move around?
Frequency	How often does it occur?
Quality	How intense is the discomfort? Is it dull, sharp, burning, throbbing, etc.?
Quantity	How long does it last?
Setting	What were you doing when it happened?
Associated findings	Are there other signs and symptoms that occur when this happens?
Aggravating and alleviating factors	What things make it worse? What things make it better?

2.6 ▶ Chest Pain Assessment

	Ask the Question:	Examples:
P (Provoke)	What provokes the pain or what precipitates the pain?	Climbing the stairs, walking; or may be unpredictable—comes on at rest.
Q (Quality)	What is the quality of the pain?	Pressure, tightness; may have associated symptoms such as nausea, vomiting, diaphoresis
R (Radiation)	Does the pain radiate to locations other than the chest?	Jaw, neck, scapular area, or left arm
S (Severity)	What is the severity of the pain (on a scale of 1 to 10)?	On a scale of 1 to 10, with 10 being the worst, how bad is your pain?
T (Timing)	What is the time of onset of this episode of pain that caused you to come to the hospital?	When did this episode of pain that brought you to the hospital start?
		Did this episode wax and wane or was it constant?
		For how many days, months, or years have you had similar pain?

2.7 ► Pain Assessment Tools for Critically Ill Patients

Numeric Rating Scales (NRS)

NRS Verbal *(0 to 10 scale)*	NRS-101 *(0 to 100 scale)*
0 = no pain	0 = no pain
10 = worst pain imaginable	100 = worst pain imaginable

Verbal Descriptive Scale

None   Mild   Moderate   Severe

Visual Analogue Scale

no pain _____ worst pain imaginable

2.8 ► Glasgow Coma Scale

Behavior	Score*
Eye Opening (E)	
Spontaneous	4
To speech	3
To pain	2
None	1
Motor Response (M)	
Obeys commands	6
Localizes pain	5
Withdraws to pain	4
Abnormal flexion	3
Extensor response	2
None	1
Verbal Response (V)	
Oriented	5
Confused	4
Inappropriate words	3
Incomprehensible sounds	2
None	1

*Coma score = E + M + V (Scores range from 3 to 15)

2.9 ▸ Glasgow Coma Scale: Motor Movement with Noxious Stimuli

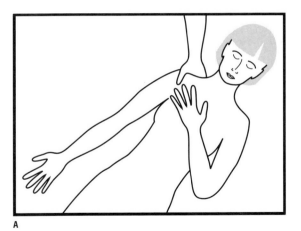

A

Localization movement toward the site of noxious stimuli (trapezius squeeze) in a quick motion.

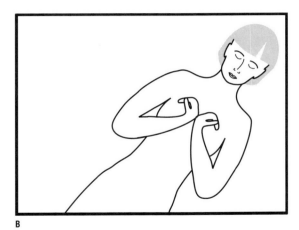

B

Decorticate posturing (into the core) is abnormal flexion with internal rotation of the upper extremities at the wrist.

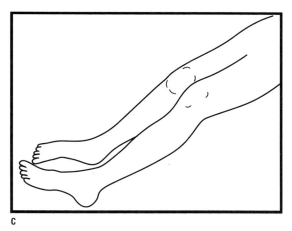

C

Lower extremity posturing is plantar flexion with internal rotation, seen with both decorticate and decerebrate posturing.

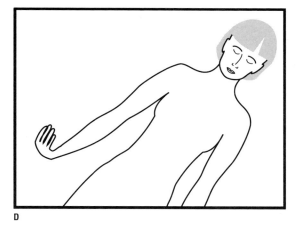

D

Decerebrate posturing is abnormal extension with external rotation of the upper extremities at the wrist.

2.10 ▸ Sensory Dermatomes

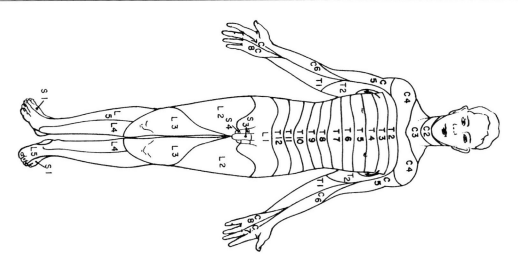

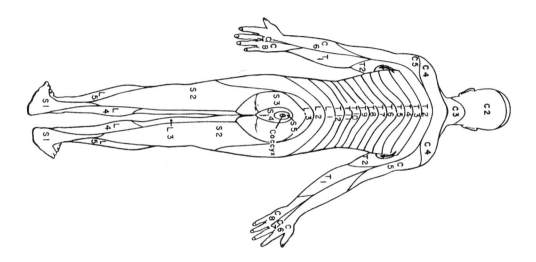

2.11 ► Peripheral Pulse Rating Scale

- 0   Absent pulse

- +1   Palpable but thready; easily obliterated with light pressure

- +2   Normal; cannot obliterate with light pressure

- +3   Full

- +4   Full and bounding

2.12 ▶ Edema Rating Scale

Following the application and removal of firm digital pressure against the tissue, the edema is evaluated for one of the following responses:

- 0   No depression in tissue

- +1   Small depression in tissue, disappearing in less than 1 second

- +2   Depression in tissue disappears in less than 1 to 2 seconds

- +3   Depression in tissue disappears in less than 2 to 3 seconds

- +4   Depression in tissue disappears in 4 seconds or longer

2.13 ► Physiologic Effects of Aging

Body System	Effects
Nervous	Diminished hearing and vision, short-term memory loss, altered motor coordination, decreased muscle tone and strength, slower response to verbal and motor stimuli, decreased ability to synthesize new information, increased sensitivity to altered temperature states, increased sensitivity to sedation (confusion or agitation), decreased alertness levels.
Cardiovascular	Increased effects of atherosclerosis of vessels and heart valves, decreased stroke volume with resulting decreased cardiac output, decreased myocardial compliance, increased workload of heart, diminished peripheral pulses.
Respiratory	Decreased compliance and elasticity, decreased vital capacity, increased residual volume, less effective cough, decreased response to hypercapnia.
Renal	Decreased glomerular filtration rate, increased risk of fluid and electrolyte imbalances.
Gastrointestinal	Increased presence of dentation problems, decreased intestinal mobility, decreased hepatic metabolism, increased risk of altered nutritional states.
Endocrine, Hematologic, and Immunologic	Increased incidence of diabetes, thyroid disorders, and anemia; decreased antibody response and cellular immunity.
Integumentary	Decreased skin turgor, increased capillary fragility and bruising, decreased elasticity.
Miscellaneous	Altered pharmacokinetics and pharmacodynamics, decreased range of motion of joints and extremities.
Psychosocial	Difficulty falling asleep and fragmented sleep patterns, increased incidence of depression and anxiety, cognitive impairment disorders, difficulty with change.

Cardiovascular System

3.1 ► ECG Lead Placement for a Three-Wire System

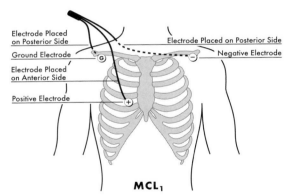

Electrode Placed on Posterior Side
Ground Electrode
Electrode Placed on Anterior Side
Positive Electrode
Electrode Placed on Posterior Side
Negative Electrode

MCL₁

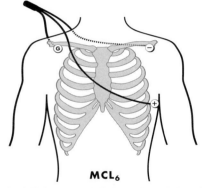

MCL₆

Lead MCL₁: ground electrode on the posterior right shoulder, negative electrode on the posterior left shoulder, and positive electrode in the V₁ position (fourth intercostal space, right of the sternum).

Lead MCL₆: ground electrode on the posterior right shoulder, negative electrode on the posterior left shoulder, and positive electrode in the V₆ position (horizontal from V₄ in the midaxillary line).

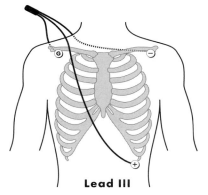

Lead III

Lead III: the positive electrode is placed on the upper left abdomen.

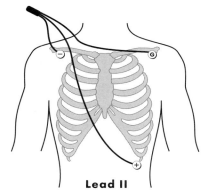

Lead II

Lead II: ground electrode on the left shoulder, negative electrode on right shoulder, and positive electrode on the left lower rib cage.

3.2 ► ECG Lead Placement for a Five-Wire System

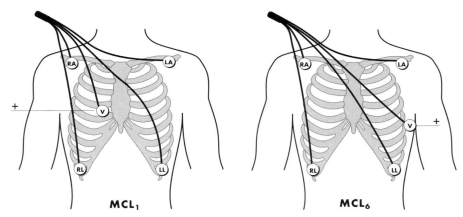

MCL₁   **MCL₆**

Electrodes are placed on the right and left shoulders, right and left lower chest areas, and in the V_1 or V_6 position. Selection of leads is made on the bedside monitor control panel.

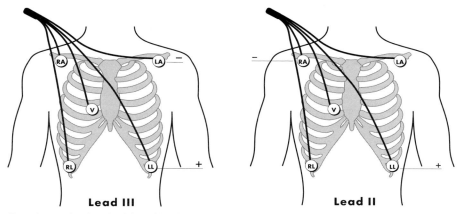

Lead III   **Lead II**

Electrodes are placed on the right and left shoulders, right and left lower chest areas, and in the V_1 or V_6 position. Selection of leads is made on the bedside monitor control panel.

3.3 ► Twelve-Lead ECG Placement

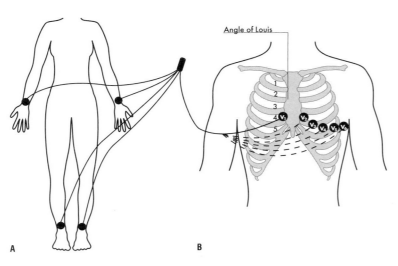

Angle of Louis

A

B

(A) Limb electrodes can be placed anywhere on arms and legs. Standard placement is shown here on wrists and ankles.

(B) Chest electrode placement. V_1 = fourth intercostal space to right of sternum; V_2 = fourth intercostal space to left of sternum; V_3 = halfway between V_2 and V_4 in a straight line; V_4 = fifth intercostal space at midclavicular line; V_5 = same level as V_4 at anterior axillary line; V_6 = same level as V_4 at midaxillary line.

3.4 ► Recommended Leads for Continuous ECG Monitoring

Purpose	Best Leads
Arrhythmia detection	V_1 or MCL_1 (V_6 or MCL_6 next best)
RCA ischemia, inferior MI	III, AVF
LAD ischemia, anterior MI	V_2, V_3, V_4 (III, aVF best limb leads)
Circumflex ischemia, lateral MI	III, aVF, V_2
RV infarction	V_4R
Wellens warning	V_2 or V_3
Axis shifts	I and aVF together

3.5 ► Cardiac Rhythms, ECG Characteristics, and Treatment Guide

Rhythm	ECG Characteristics	Treatment
Normal sinus rhythm (NSR)	• Rate: 60 to 100 beats/minute • Rhythm: Regular • P waves: Precede every QRS; consistent shape • PR interval: 0.12 to 0.20 second • QRS complex: 0.04 to 0.10 second	• None

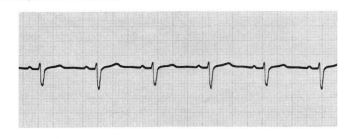

Rhythm	ECG Characteristics	Treatment
Sinus bradycardia	• Rate: Less than 60 beats/minute • Rhythm: Regular • P waves: Precede every QRS; consistent shape • PR interval: Usually normal (0.12 to 0.20 second) • QRS complex: Usually normal (0.04 to 0.10 second) • Conduction: Normal through atria, AV node, bundle branches, and ventricles	• Treat only if symptomatic • Atropine 0.5 to 1.0 mg IV

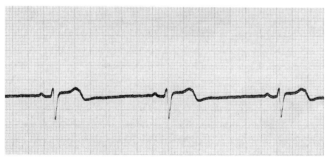

3.5 ► Cardiac Rhythms, ECG Characteristics, and Treatment Guide *(continued)*

Rhythm	ECG Characteristics	Treatment
Sinus tachycardia	• Rate: Greater than 100 beats/minute • Rhythm: Regular • P waves: Precede every QRS; consistent shape • PR interval: Usually normal (0.12 to 0.20 second); may be difficult to measure if P waves are buried in T waves • QRS complex: Usually normal (0.04 to 0.10 second) • Conduction: Normal through atria, AV node, bundle branches, and ventricles	• Treat underlying cause

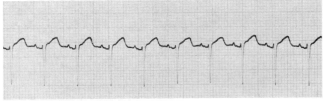

Rhythm	ECG Characteristics	Treatment
Sinus arrhythmia	• Rate: 60 to 100 beats/minute • Rhythm: Irregular; phasic increase and decrease in rate, which may or may not be related to respiration • P waves: Precede every QRS; consistent shape • PR interval: Usually normal • QRS complex: Usually normal • Conduction: Normal through atria, AV node, bundle branches, and ventricles	• Treatment usually not required • Hold digoxin if due to digitalis toxicity

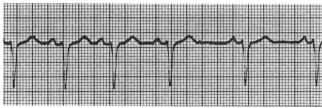

3.5 ► Cardiac Rhythms, ECG Characteristics, and Treatment Guide *(continued)*

Rhythm	ECG Characteristics	Treatment
Sinus arrest	• Rate: Usually within normal range, but may be in the bradycardia range • Rhythm: Irregular due to absence of sinus node discharge • P waves: Present when sinus node is firing and absent during periods of sinus arrest. When present, they precede every QRS complex and are consistent in shape. • PR interval: Usually normal when P waves are present • QRS complex: Usually normal when sinus node is functioning and absent during periods of sinus arrest, unless escape beats occur • Conduction: Normal through atria, AV node, bundle branches, and ventricles when sinus node is firing. When the sinus node fails to form impulses, there is no conduction through the atria.	• Treat underlying cause • Discontinue drugs that may be causative • Minimize vagal stimulation • For frequent sinus arrest causing hemodynamic compromise, atropine 0.5 to 1.0 mg IV may increase heart rate • Pacemaker may be necessary for refractory cases

Sinus arrest

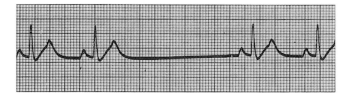

3.5 ▶ Cardiac Rhythms, ECG Characteristics, and Treatment Guide *(continued)*

Rhythm	ECG Characteristics	Treatment
Premature atrial contraction	• Rate: Usually within normal range • Rhythm: Usually regular except when PACs occur, resulting in early beats. PACs usually have a noncompensatory pause. • P waves: Precede every QRS. The configuration of the premature P wave differs from that of the sinus P waves. • PR interval: May be normal or long depending on the prematurity of the beat. Very early PACs may find the AV junction still partially refractory and unable to conduct at a normal rate, resulting in a prolonged PR interval. • QRS complex: May be normal, aberrant (wide), or absent, depending on the prematurity of the beat • Conduction: PACs travel through the atria differently from sinus impulses because they originate from a different spot. Conduction through the AV node, bundle branches, and ventricles is usually normal unless the PAC is very early.	• Treatment usually not necessary • Treat underlying cause • Drugs (e.g., quinidine, disopyramide, procainamide) can be used if necessary

**PAC conducted
normally in
ventricle**

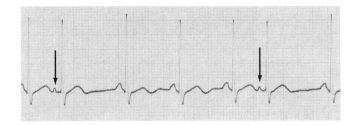

**PAC conducted
abnormally in
ventricle**

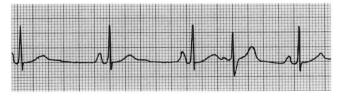

3.5 ▶ Cardiac Rhythms, ECG Characteristics, and Treatment Guide *(continued)*

Rhythm	ECG Characteristics	Treatment
Wandering atrial pacemaker	• Rate: 60 to 100 beats/minute. If the rate is faster than 100 beats/minute, it is called multifocal atrial tachycardia (MAT). • Rhythm: May be slightly irregular • P waves: Varying shapes (upright, flat, inverted, notched) as impulses originate in different parts of the atria or junction. At least three different P-wave shapes should be seen. • PR interval: May vary depending on proximity of the pacemaker to the AV node • QRS complex: Usually normal • Conduction: Conduction through the atria varies as they are depolarized from different spots. Conduction through the bundle branches and ventricles is usually normal.	• Treatment usually not necessary • Treat underlying cause • For symptoms from slow rate can use atropine • With rate >100, drugs to decrease atrial ectopy (e.g., quinidine) and/or slow ventricular rate (e.g., verapamil, propranolol) may be necessary

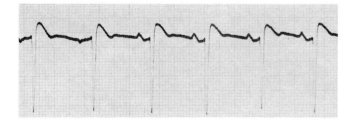

Rhythm	ECG Characteristics	Treatment
Atrial tachycardia	• Rate: Atrial rate is 150 to 250 beats/minute. • Rhythm: Regular unless there is variable block at the AV node • P waves: Differ in shape from sinus P waves because they are ectopic. Precede each QRS complex but may be hidden in preceding T wave. When block is present, more than one P wave will appear before each QRS complex. • PR interval: May be shorter than normal but often difficult to measure because of hidden P waves • QRS complex: Usually normal but may be wide if aberrant conduction is present • Conduction: Usually normal through the AV node and into the ventricles. In atrial tachycardia with block some atrial impulses do not conduct into the ventricles. Aberrant ventricular conduction may occur if atrial impulses are conducted into the ventricles while the ventricles are still partially refractory.	• Eliminate underlying cause and decrease ventricular rate • Sedation • Vagal stimulation • Vasopressors • Digitalis (unless it is the cause of atrial tachycardia with block) • Propranolol, verapamil, or diltiazem • Cardioversion for significant symptoms • Quinidine to prevent recurrences

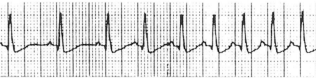

3.5 ► Cardiac Rhythms, ECG Characteristics, and Treatment Guide *(continued)*

Rhythm	ECG Characteristics	Treatment
Atrial flutter	• Rate: Atrial rate varies between 250 to 350 beats/minute, most commonly 300. Ventricular rate varies depending on the amount of block at the AV node, most commonly 150 beats/minute and rarely 300 beats/minute. • Rhythm: Atrial rhythm is regular. Ventricular rhythm may be regular or irregular due to varying AV block. • P waves: F waves (flutter waves) are seen, characterized by a very regular, "sawtooth" pattern. One F wave is usually hidden in the QRS complex, and when 2:1 conduction occurs, F waves may not be readily apparent. • FR interval (flutter wave to the beginning of the QRS complex): May be consistent or may vary • QRS complex: Usually normal; aberration can occur • Conduction: Usually normal through the AV node and ventricles	• Treatment depends on hemodynamic consequences of arrhythmia • Cardioversion for markedly reduced cardiac output • Verapamil, diltiazem, or propranolol to slow ventricular rate • Quinidine or procainamide ONLY after prior treatment to ensure adequate AV block

Atrial flutter with 4:1 conduction

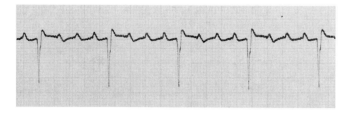

Atrial flutter with 2:1 conduction

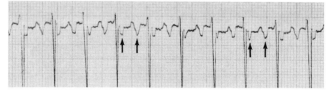

3.5 ▶ Cardiac Rhythms, ECG Characteristics, and Treatment Guide *(continued)*

Rhythm	ECG Characteristics	Treatment
Atrial fibrillation	• Rate: Atrial rate is 400 to 600 beats/minute or faster. Ventricular rate varies depending on the amount of block at the AV node. In new atrial fibrillation, the ventricular response is usually quite rapid, 160 to 200 beats/minute; in treated atrial fibrillation, the ventricular rate is controlled in the normal range of 60 to 100 beats/minute. • Rhythm: Irregular. One of the distinguishing features of atrial fibrillation is the marked irregularity of the ventricular response. • P waves: Not present. Atrial activity is chaotic with no formed atrial impulses visible. Irregular F waves are often seen and vary in size from coarse to very fine. • PR interval: Not measurable since there are no P waves • QRS complex: Usually normal; aberration is common • Conduction: Conduction within the atria is disorganized and follows a very irregular pattern. Most of the atrial impulses are blocked within the AV junction. Those impulses that are conducted through the AV junction are usually conducted normally through the ventricles. If an atrial impulse reaches the bundle branch system during its refractory period, aberrant intraventricular conduction can occur.	• Eliminate underlying cause, decrease atrial irritability, and decrease ventricular rate • Digitalis, verapamil, diltiazem, or propranolol to decrease ventricular rate • Quinidine, procainamide, flecainide, or amiodarone to decrease atrial irritability • Cardioversion for hemodynamic instability

Atrial fibrillation with controlled ventricular response

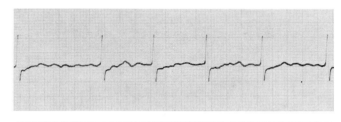

Atrial fibrillation with uncontrolled ventricular response

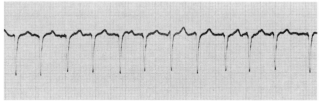

3.5 ▶ Cardiac Rhythms, ECG Characteristics, and Treatment Guide *(continued)*

Rhythm	ECG Characteristics	Treatment
Premature junctional complexes	• Rate: 60 to 100 beats/minute or whatever the rate of the basic rhythm • Rhythm: Regular except for occurrence of premature beats • P waves: May occur before, during, or after the QRS complex of the premature beat and are usually inverted • PR interval: Short, usually 0.10 second or less, when P waves precede the QRS • QRS complex: Usually normal but may be aberrant if the PJC occurs very early and conducts into the ventricles during the refractory period of a bundle branch • Conduction: Retrograde through the atria; usually normal through the ventricles	• Treatment usually not necessary • Quinidine or procainamide sometimes used

**Premature
junctional complex**

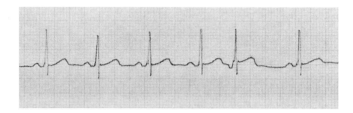

3.5 ► Cardiac Rhythms, ECG Characteristics, and Treatment Guide *(continued)*

Rhythm	ECG Characteristics	Treatment
Junctional rhythm	• Rate: Junctional rhythm, 40 to 60 beats/minute; accelerated junctional rhythm, 60 to 100 beats/minute; junctional tachycardia, 100 to 250 beats/minute • Rhythm: Regular • P waves: May precede or follow QRS • PR interval: Short, 0.11 second or less if P waves precede QRS • QRS complex: Usually normal • Conduction: Retrograde through the atria; normal through the ventricles	• Treatment rarely needed unless rate too slow or too fast to maintain adequate cardiac output • Atropine used to increase rate • Verapamil, propranolol, quinidine, or digitalis used to decrease rate • Cardioversion for rapid rate with severely reduced cardiac output • Withhold digitalis if digitalis toxicity suspected

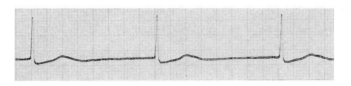

**Accelerated
junctional rhythm**

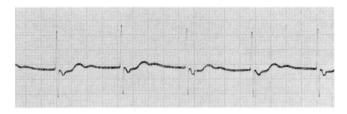

**Junctional
tachycardia**

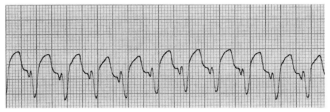

3.5 ▶ Cardiac Rhythms, ECG Characteristics, and Treatment Guide *(continued)*

Rhythm	ECG Characteristics	Treatment
Premature ventricular complexes	• Rate: 60 to 100 beats/minute or the rate of the basic rhythm • Rhythm: Irregular because of the early beats • P waves: Not related to the PVCs. Sinus rhythm is usually not interrupted by the premature beats, so sinus P waves can often be seen occurring regularly throughout the rhythm. • PR interval: Not present before most PVCs. If a P wave happens, by coincidence, to precede a PVC, the PR interval is short. • QRS complex: Wide and bizare; greater than 0.10 second in duration. May vary in morphology (size, shape) if they originate from more than one focus in the ventricles. • Conduction: Wide QRS complexes. Some PVCs may conduct retrograde into the atria, resulting in inverted P waves following the PVC.	• Eliminate underlying cause • Acute treatment with lidocaine, procainamide, or bretylium IV • Disopyramide, quinidine, propranolol, amiodarone, tocainide, mexiletine, or sotalol for long-term control

**Premature
ventricular complex**

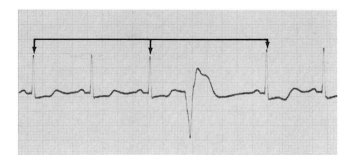

3.5 ▶ Cardiac Rhythms, ECG Characteristics, and Treatment Guide *(continued)*

Rhythm	ECG Characteristics	Treatment
Ventricular rhythm	• Rate: Less than 50 beats/minute for ventricular rhythm and 50 to 100 beats/minute for accelerated ventricular rhythm • Rhythm: Usually regular • P waves: May be seen but at a slower rate than the ventricular focus, with dissociation from the QRS • PR interval: Not measured • QRS complex: Wide and bizarre • Conduction: If sinus rhythm is the basic rhythm, atrial conduction is normal. Impulses originating in the ventricles conduct via muscle cell-to-cell conduction, resulting in the wide QRS complex.	• Treatment of accelerated ventricular rhythm only if symptomatic (e.g., with suppressive therapy as for VT) • For ventricular escape rhythms, increase rate or use temporary pacemaker

Escape ventricular rhythm

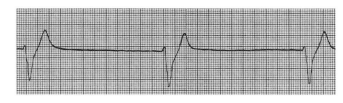

Accelerated ventricular rhythm

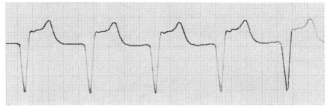

3.5 ► Cardiac Rhythms, ECG Characteristics, and Treatment Guide *(continued)*

Rhythm	ECG Characteristics	Treatment
Ventricular tachycardia	• Rate: Ventricular rate is faster than 100 beats/minute • Rhythm: Usually regular but may be slightly irregular • P waves: P waves may be seen but will not be related to QRS complexes (dissociated from QRS complexes). If sinus rhythm is the underlying basic rhythm, regular. P waves are often buried within QRS complexes. • PR interval: Not measurable because of dissociation of P waves from QRS complexes • QRS complex: Wide and bizarre; greater than 0.10 second in duration • Conduction: Impulse originates in one ventricle and spreads via muscle cell-to-cell conduction through both ventricles. There may be retrograde conduction through the atria, but more often the sinus node continues to fire regularly and depolarize the atria normally.	• Treatment depends on how rhythm is tolerated • Lidocaine, procainamide, bretylium, or magnesium sulfate for patients without severe symtoms • Cardioversion preferred (defibrillation OK) for severely symptomatic VT • CPR required for pulseless VT • Prevent recurrences with drugs used for PVCs

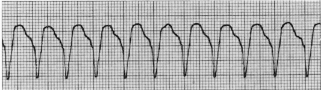

Rhythm	ECG Characteristics	Treatment
Ventricular fibrillation	• Rate: Rapid, uncoordinated, ineffective • Rhythm: Chaotic, irregular • P waves: None seen • PR interval: None • QRS complex: No formed QRS complexes seen; rapid, irregular undulations without any specific pattern • Conduction: Multiple ectopic foci firing simultaneously in ventricles and depolarizing them irregularly and without any organized pattern. Ventricles are not contracting.	• Immediate defibrillation • CPR required until defibrillator available • Lidocaine, procainamide, magnesium sulfate, or bretylium commonly used adjuncts • Epinephrine used to convert fine VF to coarser VF • After conversion of rhythm, use IV antiarrhythmics to prevent recurrence

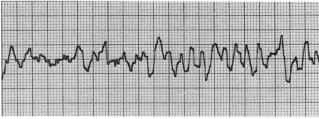

3.5 ► Cardiac Rhythms, ECG Characteristics, and Treatment Guide *(continued)*

Rhythm	ECG Characteristics	Treatment
Ventricular asystole	• Rate: None • Rhythm: None • P waves: May be present if the sinus node is functioning • PR interval: None • QRS complex: None • Conduction: Atrial conduction may be normal if the sinus node is functioning. There is no conduction into the ventricles.	• Immediate CPR • IV epinephrine • Atropine • Pacemaker

Rhythm	ECG Characteristics	Treatment
First-degree AV block	• Rate: Can occur at any sinus rate, usually 60 to 100 beats/minute • Rhythm: Regular • P waves: Normal; precede every QRS • PR interval: Prolonged above 0.20 second • QRS complex: Usually normal • Conduction: Normal through the atria, usually delayed through the AV node. Ventricular conduction is normal.	• Treatment usually not necessary

3.5 ▶ Cardiac Rhythms, ECG Characteristics, and Treatment Guide *(continued)*

Rhythm	ECG Characteristics	Treatment
Second-degree AV block type I (Wenckebach; Mobitz I)	• Rate: Can occur at any sinus or atrial rate • Rhythm: Irregular. Overall appearance of the rhythm demonstrates "group beating." • P waves: Normal. Some P waves are not conducted to the ventricles, but only one at a time fails to conduct to the ventricle. • PR interval: Gradually lengthens in consecutive beats. The PR interval preceding the pause is longer than that following the pause. • QRS complex: Usually normal unless there is associated bundle branch block • Conduction: Normal through the atria, progressively delayed through the AV node until an impulse fails. Conduction ratios can vary, with ratios as low as 2:1 (every other P wave is blocked), up to high ratios such as 15:14 (every fifteenth P wave blocked).	• Treatment depends on conduction ratio, ventricular rate, and symptoms • Atropine used for slow ventricular rate • No treatment with normal ventricular rate • Discontinue digitalis or beta blockers if suspected of causing block • Temporary pacemaker occasionally needed for slow ventricular rate

Rhythm	ECG Characteristics	Treatment
Second-degree AV block type II (Mobitz II)	• Rate: Can occur at any basic rate • Rhythm: Irregular due to blocked beats • P waves: Usually regular and precede each QRS. Periodically a P wave is not followed by a QRS complex. • PR interval: Constant before conducted beats. The PR interval preceding the pause is the same as that following the pause. • QRS complex: Usually wide due to associated bundle branch block • Conduction: Normal through the atria and through the AV node but intermittently blocked in the bundle branch system and fails to reach the ventricles. Conduction through the ventricles is abnormally slow due to associated bundle branch block. Conduction ratios can vary from 2:1 to only occasional blocked beats.	• Pacemaker usually needed • CPR for slow rate and severely decreased cardiac output • Atropine

3.5 ► Cardiac Rhythms, ECG Characteristics, and Treatment Guide *(continued)*

Rhythm	ECG Characteristics	Treatment
High AV block	• Rate: Atrial rate less than 135 beats/minute • Rhythm: Regular or irregular, depending on conduction pattern • P waves: Normal; present before every conducted QRS, but two or more consecutive P waves may not be followed by QRS complexes • PR interval: Constant before conducted beats; may be normal or prolonged • QRS complex: Usually normal in type I and wide in type II advanced blocks • Conduction: Normal through the atria. Two or more consecutive atrial impulses fail to conduct to the ventricles. Ventricular conduction is normal in type I and abnormally slow in type II advanced blocks.	• Treatment necessary if patient symptomatic • Atropine may increase ventricular rate • Pacemaker may be required

High AV block

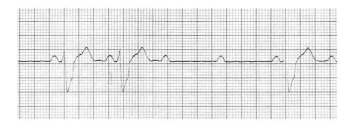

3.5 ▶ Cardiac Rhythms, ECG Characteristics, and Treatment Guide *(continued)*

Rhythm	ECG Characteristics	Treatment
Third-degree AV block	• Rate: Atrial rate is usually normal; ventricular rate is less than 45 beats/minute • Rhythm: Regular • P waves: Normal but dissociated from QRS complexes • PR interval: No consistent PR intervals because there is no relationship between P waves and QRS complexes • QRS complex: Normal if ventricles controlled by a junctional rhythm; wide if controlled by a ventricular rhythm • Conduction: Normal through the atria. All impulses are blocked at the AV node or in the bundle branches, so there is no conduction to the ventricles. Conduction through the ventricles is normal if a junctional escape rhythm occurs, and abnormally slow if a ventricular escape rhythm occurs.	• Pacemaker • Atropine usually not effective • With severely decreased cardiac output, perform CPR until pacemaker available

Third degree AV block with a junctional rhythm

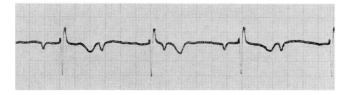

Third degree AV block with a ventricular rhythm

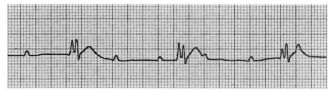

3.5 ► Cardiac Rhythms, ECG Characteristics, and Treatment Guide *(continued)*

Rhythm	ECG Characteristics	Treatment
Ventricular paced rhythm with capture	• Rate: Depends on type of pacemaker • Rhythm: Regular • P waves: Absent, or present but dissociated from QRS complexes • PR interval: None • QRS complex: Pacemaker spike followed immediately by wide, bizarre QRS complex	• None

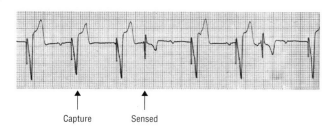

        Capture   Sensed

Rhythm	ECG Characteristics	Treatment
Ventricular paced rhythm without capture	• Conduction: Abnormal • ECG characteristics depend on nature of intrinsic rhythm • Pacemaker spike has no fixed relationship to QRS complexes	• If hemodynamically stable, elective correction/replacement of pacemaker • If hemodynamically unstable, treatment as for third-degree AV block

Ventricular spikes

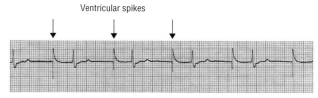

3.6 ► Normal Twelve-Lead ECG Waves

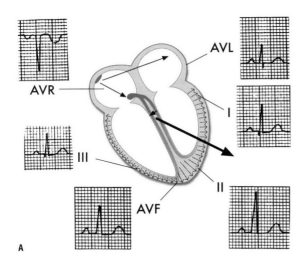

AVL

AVR

I

III

II

AVF

(A) Normal sequence of depolarization through the heart as recorded by each of the frontal plane leads.

A

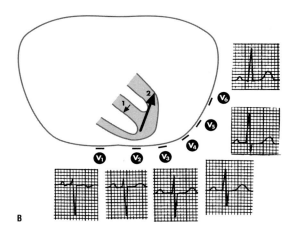

B

(B) Cross section of the thorax illustrating how the six precordial leads record normal electrical activity in the ventricles. The small arrow (1) shows the initial direction of depolarization through the septum, followed by the direction of ventricular depolarization, indicated by the larger arrow (2).

3.7 ► Normal ST Segment and T Waves

Lead II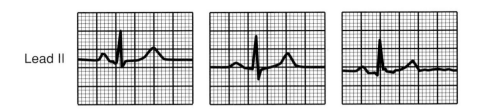

Lead V$_I$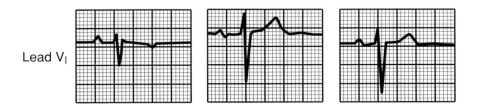

3.8 ► Zones of Myocardial Ischemia, Injury, and Infarction with Associated ECG Changes

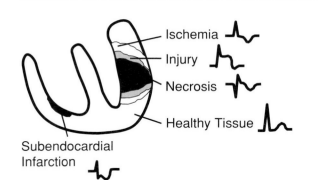

Ischemia

Injury

Necrosis

Healthy Tissue

Subendocardial Infarction

A

(A) Indicative changes seen in leads facing the injured area.

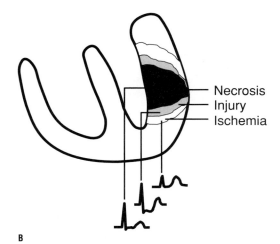

Necrosis
Injury
Ischemia

(B) Reciprocal changes often seen in leads not directly facing the involved area.

B

3.9 ► ECG Patterns Associated with Myocardial Ischemia

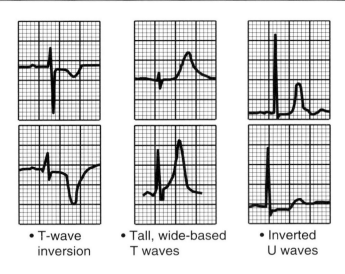

- T-wave inversion
- Tall, wide-based T waves
- Inverted U waves

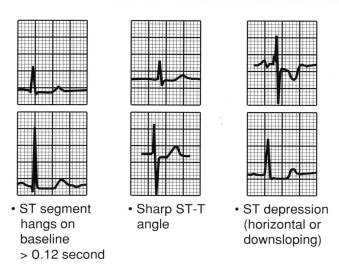

- ST segment hangs on baseline > 0.12 second

- Sharp ST-T angle

- ST depression (horizontal or downsloping)

3.10 ► ECG Patterns Associated with Acute Myocardial Injury

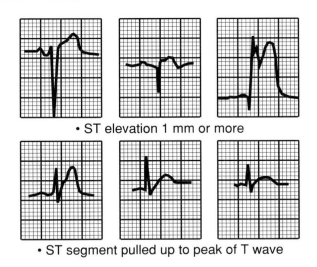

• ST elevation 1 mm or more

• ST segment pulled up to peak of T wave

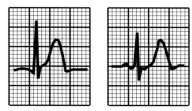

• Tall, peaked T waves

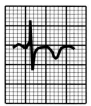

• Symmetrical T inversion

3.11 ► ECG Changes Associated with Myocardial Infarction

Location of MI	Indicative Changes	Reciprocal Changes
Anterior	V_1 to V_4	I, aVL, II, III, aVF
Septal	V_1, V_2	I, aVL
Inferior	II, III, aVF	I, aVL, V_1 to V_4
Posterior	None	V_1 to V_4
Lateral	I, aVL, V_5, V_6	II, III, aVF, V_1, V_2
Right ventricle	V_3R to V_6R	

Type MI (Arterial Involvement)	Muscle Area Supplied	Assessment	ECG Changes	Likely Dysrhythmias	Possible Complications
Anteroseptal wall (LAD)	Anterior LV wall, Anterior LV septum Apex LV Bundle of His Bundle branches	↓ LV Function → ↓ CO, ↓ BP ↑ PAD, ↑ PCWP S_3 and S_4, with CHF Rales with pulmonary edema	**Indicative:** ST elevation with or without abnormal Q waves in $V_{1,2,3,4}$ Loss of R waves in precordial leads **Reciprocal:** ST depression in II, III, AVF	RBBB, LBBB AV blocks Atrial fibrillation or flutter Ventricular tachycardia (VT) Tachycardia (septal)	Cardiogenic shock VSD Myocardial rupture Heart blocks may be permanent (LBBB) High mortality associated with this location of MI

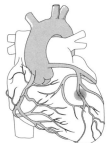

3.12 ► Clinical Presentation of Myocardial Ischemia and Infarction *(continued)*

Type MI (Arterial Involvement)	Muscle Area Supplied	Assessment	ECG Changes	Likely Dysrhythmias	Possible Complications
Posterior septal lateral (RCA)	Posterior surface of LV SA node 45% AV node 10% Left atrium Lateral wall of LV	Murmurs indicating VSD (septal) PA catheter to assess R to L shunt in VSD Signs/symptoms of LV aneurysm with lateral Displaced PMI leading to signs and symptoms of mitral regurgitation	**Lateral Indicative:** ST elevation I, AVL, $V_{5,6}$ Loss of R wave and ↑ ST in I, AVL, $V_{5,6}$ **Posterior Indicative:** Tall, broad R waves (>0.04 sec) in V_{1-3} ↑ ST V_4R (right-sided 12-lead, V_4 position) **Posterior Reciprocal:** ST depression in $V_{1,2}$, upright T wave in $V_{1,2}$	Bradycardia Mobitz I (posterior)	RV involvement Aneurysm development Papillary muscle dysfunction Heart blocks frequently resolve

Type MI (Arterial Involvement)	Muscle Area Supplied	Assessment	ECG Changes	Likely Dysrhythmias	Possible Complications
Inferior or "diaphragmatic" (RCA)	RV, RA SA Node 50% AV Node 90% RA, RV Inferior LV Posterior IV Septum Posterior LBBB Posterior LV	Symptomatic bradycardia: ↓ BP LOC changes diaphoresis ↓ CO ↑ PAD ↑ PCWP Murmurs: associated with papillary muscle dysfunction, mid/holosystolic rales, pulmonary edema, nausea	**Indicative:** ↑ ST segments in II, III, AVF Q waves in II, III, AVF **Reciprocal:** ST depression in I, AVL, $V_{1,2,3,4}$	AV blocks; often progress to CHB which may be transient or permanent; Wenckebach; bradyarrhythmias	Hiccups Nausea/vomiting Papillary muscle dysfunction MR Septal rupture (0.5%–1%) RV involvement associated with atrial infarcts especially with atrial dysrhythmias

3.12 ► Clinical Presentation of Myocardial Ischemia and Infarction *(continued)*

Type MI (Arterial Involvement)	Muscle Area Supplied	Assessment	ECG Changes	Likely Dysrhythmias	Possible Complications
Right ventricular infarction (RCA)	RA, RV, inferior LV SA Node AV Node Posterior IV Septum	Kussmaul's sign JVD Hypotension ↑ SVR, ↓ PCWP ↑ CVP S$_3$ with noncompliant RV Clear breath sounds initially Hepatomegaly, peripheral edema, cool clammy pale skin	**Indicative:** 1- to 2-mm ST-segment elevation in V$_4$R ST- and T-wave elevation in II, III, AVF Q waves in II, III, AVF ST elevation decreases in amplitude over V$_{1-6}$	First-degree AV block Second-degree AV block, type I Incomplete RBBB Transient CHB Atrial fibrillation VT/VF	Hypotension requiring large volumes initially to maintain systemic pressure. Once RV contractility improves fluids will mobilize, possibly requiring diuresis.

3.13 ► Cardiac Axis

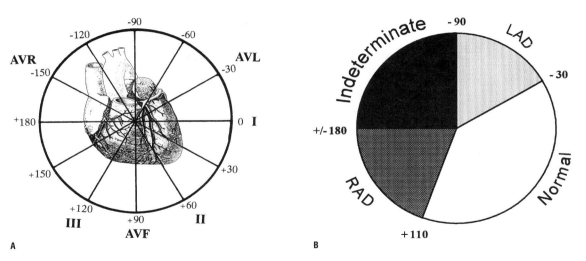

A

B

3.14 ► Causes of Axis Deviations

Axis: −30° to +110°
• Normal

Left Axis Deviation: −31° to −90°
• Left ventricular hypertrophy
• Left anterior fascicular block
• Inferior myocardial infarction
• Left bundle branch block (LBBB)
• Congenital defects
• Ventricular tachycardia
• Wolff-Parkinson-White syndrome

Right Axis Deviation: +110° to +180°
• Right ventricular hypertrophy
• Left posterior fascicular block
• Right bundle branch block (RBBB)
• Dextrocardia
• Ventricular tachycardia
• Wolff-Parkinson-White syndrome

Intermediate Axis: −90° to −180°
• Ventricular tachycardia
• Bifascicular block

3.15 ► Nomogram for Rate Correction of QT Interval

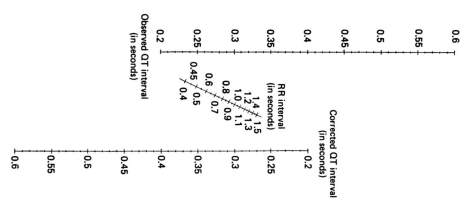

Measure the observed QT interval and the RR interval. Mark these values in the respective columns on the chart (left and middle). Place a ruler across these two points. The point at which the extension of this line crosses the third column is read as the corrected QT interval (QT$_c$). *(From: Kissen M, et al: A nomogram for rate correction of the QT interval in the electrocardiogram. American Heart Journal. 1948;35:991.)*

3.16 ► Advantages of Common ECG Monitoring Leads

Lead	Advantages
Preferred Monitoring Leads	
MCL₁ and MCL₆	Allow distinction between left ventricular and right ventricular ectopy and between left ventricular and right ventricular artificial pacing
	Allow distinction between right and left bundle branch block
	Allow distinction between aberration and ectopy
	Assist in diagnoses that require well-formed P waves
	Apex of the heart is not covered by an electrode and is clear for auscultation and defibrillation without electrode interference
Other Monitoring Leads	
M₃	Allows identification of retrograde P waves
II	Assists in the diagnosis of hemiblock

(From: Osguthorpe SG, Woods SL: Myocardial ischemia and infarction. In Woods SL, et al (eds.): Cardiac nursing, *3rd ed. Philadelphia: JB Lippincott, 1995, p 479.)*

3.17 ► Pacemaker Codes

First Letter: Chamber Paced	Second Letter: Chamber Sensed	Third Letter: Response to Sensing	Fourth Letter: Programmability, Rate Modulation	Fifth Letter: Antitachycardia Pacing Functions
O = None	O = None	O = None	O = None	O = None
A = Atrium	A = Atrium	I = Inhibited	P = Simple programmable	P = Pacing (Antitachycardia)
V = Ventricle	V = Ventricle	T = Triggered	M = Multiprogrammable	S = Shock
D = Dual (A&V)	D = Dual (A&V)	D = Dual (I&T)	C = Communicating	D = Dual (P&S)
			R = Rate modulation	

3.18 ► Dual-Chamber Pacing Modes

Mode	Chamber(s) Paced	Chamber(s) Sensed	Response to Sensing
DVI	Atrium and ventricle	Ventricle	Inhibited
VDD	Ventricle	Atrium and ventricle	Atrial sensing triggers ventricular pacing
			Ventricular sensing inhibits ventricular pacing
DDI	Atrium and ventricle	Atrium and ventricle	Inhibited
DDD	Atrium and ventricle	Atrium and ventricle	Atrial sensing inhibits atrial pacing, triggers ventricular pacing
			Ventricular sensing inhibits atrial and ventricular pacing

3.19 ▶ Intraaortic Balloon Pump Frequency of 1 : 2

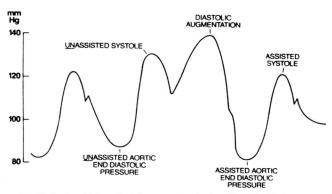

(Datascope Corporation: Mechanics of intraaortic balloon counterpulsation. Montvale, NJ: Datascope, 1989.)

3.20 ► Intraaortic Balloon Pump Frequency of 1:1

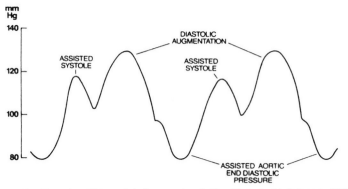

(Datascope Corporation: Mechanics of intraaortic balloon counterpulsation. Montvale, NJ: Datascope, 1989.)

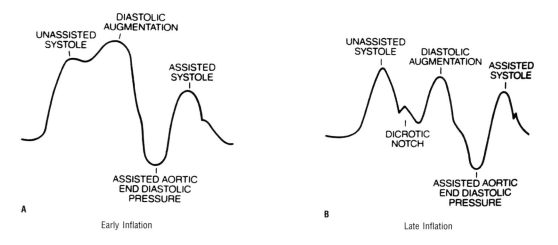

A

Early Inflation

B

Late Inflation

3.21 ► Inaccurate IABP Timing *(continued)*

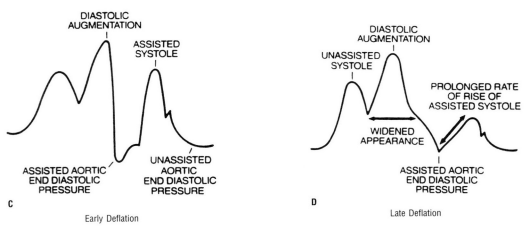

DIASTOLIC
AUGMENTATION

ASSISTED
SYSTOLE

ASSISTED AORTIC
END DIASTOLIC
PRESSURE

UNASSISTED
AORTIC
END DIASTOLIC
PRESSURE

C

Early Deflation

UNASSISTED
SYSTOLE

DIASTOLIC
AUGMENTATION

PROLONGED RATE
OF RISE OF
ASSISTED SYSTOLE

WIDENED
APPEARANCE

ASSISTED AORTIC
END DIASTOLIC
PRESSURE

D

Late Deflation

(Datascope Corporation: Mechanics of intraaortic balloon counterpulsation. *Montvale, NJ: Datascope, 1989.)*

3.22 ▶ Universal Algorithm for Adult Emergency Cardiac Care (ECC)*

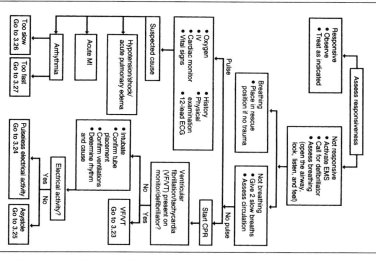

*All cardiac algorithms from: Advanced cardiac life support: Part III. Journal of the American Medical Association. 1992;268:2216.

97

3.23 ▶ Algorithm for Ventricular Fibrillation and Pulseless Ventricular Tachycardia (VF/VT)

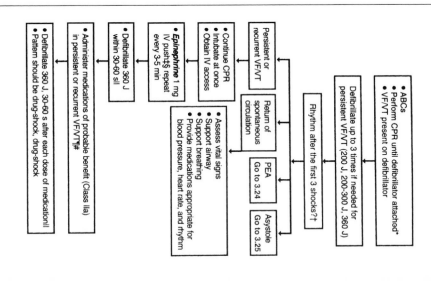

- ABCs
- Perform CPR until defibrillator attached*
- VF/VT present on defibrillator

Defibrillate up to 3 times if needed for persistent VF/VT (200 J, 200-300 J, 360 J)

Rhythm after the first 3 shocks?†

PEA
Go to 3.24

Asystole
Go to 3.25

Return of spontaneous circulation

Persistent or recurrent VF/VT

- Assess vital signs
- Support airway
- Support breathing
- Provide medications appropriate for blood pressure, heart rate, and rhythm

- Continue CPR
- Intubate at once
- Obtain IV access

• *Epinephrine* 1 mg IV push‡§ repeat every 3-5 min

• Defibrillate 360 J within 30-60 s‖

• Administer medications of probable benefit (Class IIa) in persistent or recurrent VF/VT¶#

• Defibrillate 360 J, 30-60 s after each dose of medication‖
• Pattern should be drug-shock, drug-shock

Class I: definitely helpful
Class IIa: acceptable, probably helpful
Class IIb: acceptable, possibly helpful
Class III: not indicated, may be harmful

*Precordial thump is a Class IIb action in witnessed arrest, no pulse, and no defibrillator immediately available.

†Hypothermic cardiac arrest is treated differently after this point. See section on hypothermia.

‡The recommended dose of *epinephrine* is 1 mg IV push every 3-5 min. If this approach fails, several Class IIb dosing regimens can be considered:
• Intermediate: *epinephrine* 2-5 mg IV push, every 3-5 min
• Escalating: *epinephrine* 1 mg-3 mg-5 mg IV push (3 min apart)
• High: *epinephrine* 0.1 mg/kg IV push, every 3-5 min

§ *Sodium bicarbonate* (1 mEq/kg) is Class I if patient has known preexisting hyperkalemia

‖Multiple sequenced shocks (200J, 200-300J, 360 J) are acceptable here (Class I), especially when medications are delayed

¶
• *Lidocaine* 1.5 mg/kg IV push. Repeat in 3-5 min to total loading dose of 3 mg/kg; then use
• *Bretylium* 5 mg/kg IV push. Repeat in 5 min at 10 mg/kg
• *Magnesium sulfate* 1-2 g IV in torsades de pointes or suspected hypomagnesemic state or severe refractory VF
• *Procainamide* 30 mg/min in refractory VF (maximum total 17 mg/kg)
• *Sodium bicarbonate* (1 mEq/kg IV):
Class IIa
• if known preexisting bicarbonate-responsive acidosis
• if overdose with tricyclic antidepressants
• to alkalinize the urine in drug overdoses
Class IIb
• if intubated and continued long arrest interval
• upon return of spontaneous circulation after long arrest interval
Class III
• hypoxic lactic acidosis

3.24 ▶ Algorithm for Pulseless Electrical Activity (PEA) (Electromechanical Dissociation [EMD])

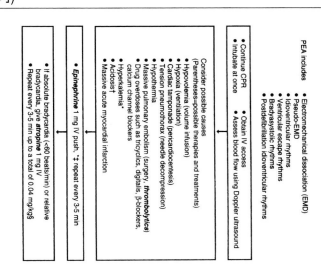

PEA includes
- Electromechanical dissociation (EMD)
- Pseudo-EMD
- Idioventricular rhythms
- Ventricular escape rhythms
- Bradyasystolic rhythms
- Postdefibrillation idioventricular rhythms

- Continue CPR
- Intubate at once
- Obtain IV access
- Assess blood flow using Doppler ultrasound

Consider possible causes
(Parentheses=possible therapies and treatments)
- Hypovolemia (volume infusion)
- Hypoxia (ventilation)
- Cardiac tamponade (pericardiocentesis)
- Tension pneumothorax (needle decompression)
- Hypothermia
- Massive pulmonary embolism (surgery, *thrombolytics*)
- Drug overdoses such as tricyclics, digitalis, β-blockers, calcium channel blockers
- Hyperkalemia*
- Acidosis†
- Massive acute myocardial infarction

- *Epinephrine* 1 mg IV push; ‡ repeat every 3-5 min

- If absolute bradycardia (<60 beats/min) or relative bradycardia, give *atropine* 1 mg IV
- Repeat every 3-5 min up to a total of 0.04 mg/kg§

Class I: definitely helpful
Class IIa: acceptable, probably helpful
Class IIb: acceptable, possibly helpful
Class III: not indicated, may be harmful

Sodium bicarbonate 1 mEq/kg is Class I if patient has known preexisting hyperkalemia.

†*Sodium bicarbonate* 1 mEq/kg:
Class IIa
● if known preexisting bicarbonate-responsive acidosis
● if overdose with tricyclic antidepressants
● to alkalinize the urine in drug overdoses
Class IIb
● if intubated and long arrest interval
● upon return of spontaneous circulation after long arrest interval
Class III
● hypoxic lactic acidosis

‡The recommended dose of *epinephrine* is 1 mg IV push every 3-5 min. If this approach fails, several Class IIb dosing regimens can be considered.
● Intermediate: *epinephrine* 2-5 mg IV push, every 3-5 min
● Escalating: *epinephrine* 1 mg-3 mg-5 mg IV push (3 min apart)
● High: *epinephrine* 0.1 mg/kg IV push, every 3-5 min

§Shorter *atropine* dosing intervals are possibly helpful in cardiac arrest (Class IIb).

101

3.25 ► Asystole Treatment Algorithm

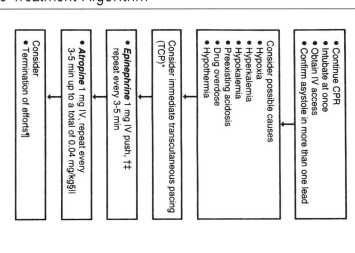

- Continue CPR
- Intubate at once
- Obtain IV access
- Confirm asystole in more than one lead

→

- Consider possible causes
  - Hypoxia
  - Hyperkalemia
  - Hypokalemia
  - Preexisting acidosis
  - Drug overdose
  - Hypothermia

→

Consider immediate transcutaneous pacing (TCP)*

→

- *Epinephrine* 1 mg IV push, †‡ repeat every 3-5 min

→

- *Atropine* 1 mg IV, repeat every 3-5 min up to a total of 0.04 mg/kg§||

→

- Consider
  - Termination of efforts¶

Class I: definitely helpful
Class IIa: acceptable, probably helpful
Class IIb: acceptable, possibly helpful
Class III: not indicated, may be harmful

*TCP is a Class IIb intervention. Lack of success may be due to delays in pacing. To be effective TCP must be performed early, simultaneously with drugs. Evidence does not support routine use of TCP for asystole.

†The recommended dose of *epinephrine* is 1 mg IV push every 3-5 min. If this approach fails, several Class IIb dosing regimens can be considered:

• Intermediate: *epinephrine* 2-5 mg IV push, every 3-5 min
• Escalating: *epinephrine* 1 mg-3 mg-5 mg IV push (3 min apart)
• High: *epinephrine* 0.1 mg/kg IV push, every 3-5 min

‡*Sodium bicarbonate* 1 mEq/kg is Class I if patient has known preexisting hyperkalemia.

§Shorter *atropine* dosing intervals are Class IIb in asystolic arrest.

‖*Sodium bicarbonate* 1 mEq/kg:
   Class IIa
   • if known preexisting bicarbonate-responsive acidosis
   • if overdose with tricyclic antidepressants
   • to alkalinize the urine in drug overdoses
   Class IIb
   • if intubated and continued long arrest interval
   • upon return of spontaneous circulation after long arrest interval
   Class III
   • hypoxic lactic acidosis

¶If patient remains in asystole or other agonal rhythms after successful intubation and initial medications and no reversible causes are identified, consider termination of resuscitative efforts by a physician. Consider interval since arrest.

3.26 ► Bradycardia Algorithm (with the Patient Not in Cardiac Arrest)

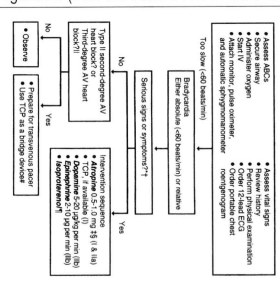

- Assess ABCs
- Secure airway
- Administer oxygen
- Start IV
- Attach monitor, pulse oximeter, and automatic sphygmomanometer

- Assess vital signs
- Review history
- Perform physical examination
- Order 12-lead ECG
- Order portable chest roentgenogram

Too slow (<60 beats/min)

Bradycardia
Either absolute (<60 beats/min) or relative

Serious signs or symptoms?*†

No → Type II second-degree AV heart block? or Third-degree AV heart block?‖

No → • Observe

Yes → • Prepare for transvenous pacer
• Use TCP as a bridge device#

Yes → Intervention sequence
- **Atropine** 0.5-1.0 mg ‡§ (I & IIa)
- TCP, if available (I)
- **Dopamine** 5-20 µg/kg per min (IIb)
- **Epinephrine** 2-10 µg per min (IIb)
- **Isoproterenol**¶‖

*Serious signs or symptoms must be related to the slow rate. Clinical manifestations include:
symptoms (chest pain, shortness of breath, decreased level of conciousness) and
signs (low BP, shock, pulmonary congestion, CHF, acute MI).

†Do not delay TCP while awaiting IV access or for *atropine* to take effect if patient is symptomatic.

‡Denervated transplanted hearts will not respond to *atropine*. Go at once to pacing, *catecholamine* infusion, or both.

§*Atropine* should be given in repeat doses in 3-5 min up to total of 0.04 mg/kg. Consider shorter dosing intervals in severe clinical conditions. It has been suggested that atropine should be used with caution in atrioventricular (AV) block at the His-Purkinje level (type II AV block and new third-degree block with wide QRS complexes) (Class IIb).

||Never treat third-degree heart block plus ventricular escape beats with *lidocaine*.

¶*Isoproterenol* should be used, if at all, with extreme caution. At low doses it is Class IIb (possibly helpful); at higher doses it is Class III (harmful).

#Verify patient tolerance and mechanical capture. Use analgesia and sedation as needed.

3.27 ► Tachycardia Algorithm

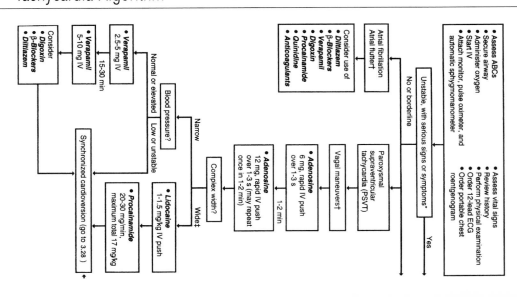

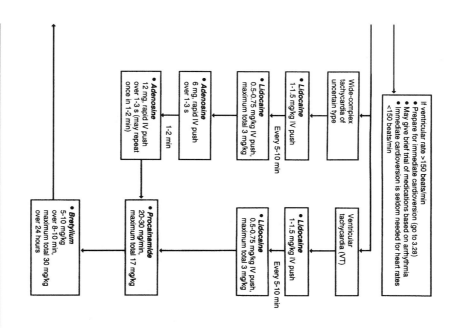

- If ventricular rate >150 beats/min
- Prepare for immediate cardioversion (go to 3.28)
- May give brief trial of medications based on arrhythmia
- Immediate cardioversion is seldom needed for heart rates <150 beats/min

Wide-complex tachycardia of uncertain type

- *Lidocaine* 1-1.5 mg/kg IV push

Every 5-10 min

- *Lidocaine* 0.5-0.75 mg/kg IV push, maximum total 3 mg/kg

- *Adenosine* 6 mg, rapid IV push over 1-3 s

1-2 min

- *Adenosine* 12 mg, rapid IV push over 1-3 s (may repeat once in 1-2 min)

Ventricular tachycardia (VT)

- *Lidocaine* 1-1.5 mg/kg IV push

Every 5-10 min

- *Lidocaine* 0.5-0.75 mg/kg IV push, maximum total 3 mg/kg

- *Procainamide* 20-30 mg/min, maximum total 17 mg/kg

- *Bretylium* 5-10 mg/kg over 8-10 min, maximum total 30 mg/kg over 24 hours

*Unstable condition must be related to the tachycardia. Signs and symptoms may include chest pain, shortness of breath, decreased level of consciousness, low blood pressure (BP), shock, pulmonary congestion, congestive heart failure, acute myocardial infarction.
†Carotid sinus pressure is contraindicated in patients with carotid bruits; avoid ice water immersion in patients with ischemic heart disease.
‡If the wide-complex tachycardia is known with certainty to be PSVT and BP is normal/elevated, sequence can include *verapamil*.

107

3.28 ► Electrical Cardioversion Algorithm (with the Patient Not in Cardiac Arrest)

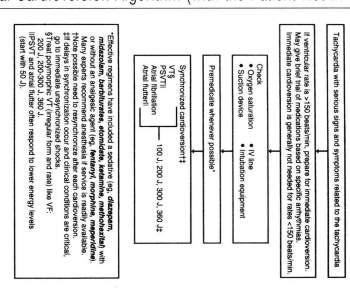

Tachycardia with serious signs and symptoms related to the tachycardia

↓

If ventricular rate is >150 beats/min, prepare for immediate cardioversion.
May give brief trial of medications based on specific arrhythmias.
Immediate cardioversion is generally not needed for rates <150 beats/min.

↓

Check
- Oxygen saturation
- Suction device
- IV line
- Intubation equipment

↓

Premedicate whenever possible*

↓

Synchronized cardioversion†‡
VT§
PSVT‖
Atrial fibrillation
Atrial flutter‖ ——— 100 J, 200 J, 300 J, 360 J‡

*Effective regimens have included a sedative (eg, **diazepam,** **midazolam, barbiturates, etomidate, ketamine, methohexital**) with or without an analgesic agent (eg, **fentanyl, morphine, meperidine**). Many experts recommend anesthesia if service is readily available.
†Note possible need to resynchronize after each cardioversion.
‡If delays in synchronization occur and clinical conditions are critical, go to immediate unsynchronized shocks.
§Treat polymorphic VT (irregular form and rate) like VF:
200 J, 200-300 J, 360 J.
‖PSVT and atrial flutter often respond to lower energy levels (start with 50 J).

3.29 ► Problems Encountered with Arterial Catheters

Problem/Cause	Prevention	Treatment
Hematoma after withdrawal of needle		
Bleeding or oozing at puncture site	Maintain firm pressure on site during withdrawal of catheter and for 5–15 minutes (as necessary) after withdrawal.	Continue to hold pressure to puncture site until oozing stops.
	Apply elastic tape (Elastoplast) firmly over puncture site.	
	For femoral arterial puncture sites, leave a sandbag on site for 1–2 hours to prevent oozing.	Apply sandbag to femoral puncture site for 1–2 hours after removal of catheter.
	If patient is receiving heparin, discontinue 2 hours before catheter removal.	
Decreased or absent pulse distal to puncture site		
Spasm of artery	Introduce arterial needle cleanly, nontraumatically.	Inject lidocaine locally at insertion site and 10 mg into arterial catheter.
Thrombosis of artery	Use 1 U heparin/1 ml IV fluid.	Arteriotomy and Fogarty catheterization both distally and proximally from the puncture site result in return of pulse in more than 90% of cases if brachial or femoral artery is used.
Bleedback into tubing, dome, or transducer		
Insufficient pressure on IV bag	Maintain 300 mm Hg pressure on IV bag.	Replace transducer. "Fast flush" through system.
Loose connections	Use Luer-Lok stopcocks; tighten periodically.	Tighten all connections.

3.29 ▶ Problems Encountered with Arterial Catheters *(continued)*

Problem/Cause	Prevention	Treatment
Hemorrhage		
Loose connections	Keep all connecting sites visible. Observe connecting sites frequently. Use built-in alarm system. Use Luer-Lok stopcocks.	Tighten all connections.
Emboli		
Clot from catheter tip into bloodstream	Always aspirate and discard before flushing. Use continuous flush device. Use 1 U heparin/1 ml IV fluid. Gently flush <2–4 ml.	Remove catheter.
Local infection		
Forward movement of contaminated catheter	Carefully suture catheter at insertion site.	Remove catheter.
Break in sterile technique Prolonged catheter use	Always use aseptic technique. Remove catheter after 72–96 hours. Leave dressing in place until catheter is removed, changed, or dressing becomes damp, loosened, or soiled.	Prescribe antibiotic.

From: Daily E, Schroeder J: Techniques in bedside hemodynamic monitoring, *5th ed. St. Louis, MO: CV Mosby, 1994, pp. 165–166.*

Problem/Cause	Prevention	Treatment
Sepsis Break in sterile technique Prolonged catheter use Bacterial growth in IV fluid	Use percutaneous insertion. Always use aseptic technique. Remove catheter after 72–96 hours. Change IV fluid bag, stopcocks, dome, and tubing no more frequently than at 72-hour intervals. Do not use IV fluid containing glucose. Use sterile dead-end caps on all ports of stopcocks. Carefully flush remaining blood from stopcocks after blood sampling.	Remove catheter. Prescribe antibiotic.

3.30 ► Inaccurate Arterial Pressure Measurements

Problem/Cause	Prevention	Treatment
Damped pressure tracing		
Catheter tip against vessel wall	Usually cannot be avoided.	Pull back, rotate, or reposition catheter while observing pressure waveform.
Partial occlusion of catheter tip by clot	Use continuous drip under pressure. Briefly "fast flush" after blood withdrawal (2–4 ml). Add 1 U heparin/1 ml IV fluid.	Aspirate clot with syringe and flush with heparinized saline (<2–4 ml).
Clot in stopcock or transducer	Carefully flush catheter after blood withdrawal and reestablish IV drip. Use continuous flush device.	Flush stopcock and transducer; if no improvement, change stopcock and transducer.
Air bubbles in transducer or connector tubing	Carefully flush transducer and tubing when setting up system and attaching to catheter.	Check system; flush rapidly; disconnect transducer and flush out air bubbles.
Compliant tubing	Use stiff, short tubing.	Shorten tubing or replace softer tubing with stiffer tubing.

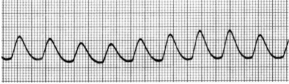

Problem/Cause	Prevention	Treatment
Abnormally high or low readings		
Change in transducer air-reference level	Maintain air-reference port of transducer at midchest and/or catheter tip level for serial pressure measurements.	Recheck patient and transducer positions.
No pressure available		
Transducer not open to catheter	Follow routine, systematic steps for setting up system and turning stopcocks.	Check system—stopcocks, monitor, and amplifier setup.
Settings on monitor amplifiers incorrect— still on zero, cal, or off		
Incorrect scale selection	Select scale appropriate to expected range of physiologic signal.	Select appropriate scale.

From: Daily E, Schroeder J: Techniques in bedside hemodynamic monitoring, *5th ed. St. Louis, MO: CV Mosby, 1994, p. 161.*

3.31 ▶ Problems Encountered with Pulmonary Artery (PA) Catheters*

Problem/Cause	Prevention	Treatment
Phlebitis or local infection at insertion site		
Mechanical irritation or contamination	Prepare skin properly before insertion. Use sterile technique during insertion and dressing change. Insert smoothly and rapidly. Use Teflon-coated introducer. Attach silver-impregnated cuff to introducer. Change dressings, stopcocks, and connecting tubing every 24–48 hours. Remove catheter or change insertion site every 4 days.	Remove catheter. Apply warm compresses. Give pain medication as necessary.
Ventricular irritability		
Looping of excess catheter in right ventricle	Suture catheter at insertion site; check chest film.	Reposition catheter; remove loop.
Migration of catheter from PA to RV	Position catheter tip in main right or left PA.	Inflate balloon to encourage catheter flotation out to PA.
Irritation of the endocardium during catheter passage	Keep balloon inflated during advancement; advance gently.	Advance rapidly out to PA.

*PAW, pulmonary artery wedge; RV, right ventricle; PA, pulmonary artery.
From Daily E, Schroeder J: Techniques in bedside hemodynamic monitoring, 5th ed. St. Louis, MO: CV Mosby, 1994, pp. 134–136.

Problem/Cause	Prevention	Treatment
Apparent wedging of catheter with balloon deflated		
Forward migration of catheter tip caused by blood flow, excessive loop in RV, or inadequate suturing of catheter at insertion site	Check catheter tip by fluoroscopy; position in main right or left PA. Check catheter position on x-ray film if fluoroscopy is not used. Suture catheter in place at insertion site.	Aspirate blood from catheter; if catheter is wedged, sample will be arterialized and obtained with difficulty.
		If wedged, slowly pull back catheter until PA waveform appears. If not wedged, gently aspirate and flush catheter with saline; catheter tip can partially clot, causing damping that resembles damped PAW waveform.

3.31 ▶ Problems Encountered with Pulmonary Artery (PA) Catheters* *(continued)*

Problem/Cause	Prevention	Treatment
Pulmonary hemorrhage or infarction, or both		
Distal migration of catheter tip	Check chest film immediately after insertion and 12–24 hrs later; remove any catheter loop in RA or RV.	Deflate balloon.
Continuous or prolonged wedging of catheter	Leave balloon deflated.	Place patient on side (catheter tip down).
	Suture catheter at skin to prevent inadvertent advancement.	Stop anticoagulation.
	Position catheter in main right or left PA.	Consider "wedge" angiogram.
	Pull catheter back to pulmonary artery if it spontaneously wedges.	
	Do not flush catheter when in wedge position.	
Overinflation of balloon while catheter is wedged	Inflate balloon slowly with only enough air to obtain a PAW waveform.	
Failure of balloon to deflate	Do not inflate 7-Fr catheter with more than 1–1.5 ml air.	

Problem/Cause	Prevention	Treatment
"Overwedging" or damped PAW		
Overinflation of balloon	Do not inflate if resistance is met.	Deflate balloon; reinflate slowly with only enough air to obtain PAW pressure.
	Watch waveform during inflation; inject only enough air to obtain PAW pressure.	Deflate balloon; reposition and slowly reinflate.
	Do not inflate 7-Fr catheter with more than 1–1.5 ml air.	
Eccentric inflation of balloon	Check inflated balloon shape before insertion.	

3.31 ▶ Problems Encountered with Pulmonary Artery (PA) Catheters* *(continued)*

Problem/Cause	Prevention	Treatment
PA balloon rupture		
Overinflation of balloon	Inflate slowly with only enough air to obtain a PAW pressure.	Remove syringe to prevent further air injection.
Frequent inflations of balloon		
Syringe deflation damaging wall of balloon	Monitor PAD pressure as reflection of PAW and LVEDP.	Monitor PAD pressure.
	Allow passive deflation of balloon.	
	Remove syringe after inflation.	
Infection		
Nonsterile insertion techniques	Use sterile techniques.	Remove catheter.
Contamination via skin	Use sterile catheter sleeve.	Use antibiotics.
	Prepare skin with effective antiseptic (chlorhexidine).	
	Leave dressing in place until catheter is removed, changed, or the dressing becomes damp, loosened, or soiled.	
	Reassess need for catheter after 3 days.	
	Avoid internal jugular approach.	
Contamination through stopcock ports or catheter hub	Use sterile dead-end caps on all stopcock ports.	
	Change tubing, continuous flush device and flush solution every 96 hours.	
	Do not use IV flush solution that contains glucose.	

Problem/Cause	Prevention	Treatment
Fluid contamination from transducer through cracked membrane of disposable dome	Check transducer domes for cracks. Change transducers every 96 hours. Change disposable dome after countershock. Do not use IV flush solution that contains glucose. Change catheter insertion site every 4 days.	
Prolonged catheter placement		
Heart block during insertion of catheter		
Mechanical irritation of His bundle in patients with preexisting left bundle branch block	Insert catheter expeditiously with balloon inflated. Insert transvenous pacing catheter before PA catheter insertion.	Use temporary pacemaker or flotation catheter with pacing wire.

3.32 ► Inaccurate Pulmonary Artery (PA) Pressure Measurements*

Problem/Cause	Prevention	Treatment
Damped waveforms and inaccurate pressures		
Partial clotting at catheter tip	Use continuous drip with 1 U heparin/1 ml IV fluid. Hand flush occasionally. Flush with large volume after blood sampling. Use heparin-coated catheters.	Aspirate, then flush catheter with heparinized fluid (not in PAW position).
Tip moving against wall	Obtain more stable catheter position.	Reposition catheter.
Kinking of catheter	Restrict catheter movement at insertion site.	Reposition to straighten catheter. Replace catheter.

*PAW, pulmonary artery wedge; RV, right ventricle; PA, pulmonary artery.
From Daily E, Schroeder J: Techniques in bedside hemodynamic monitoring, 5th ed. St. Louis, MO: CV Mosby, 1994, p. 137.

Problem/Cause	Prevention	Treatment
Abnormally low or negative pressures		
Incorrect air reference level (above midchest level)	Maintain transducer air-reference port at midchest level; rezero after patient position changes.	Remeasure level of transducer air reference and reposition at midchest level; rezero.
Incorrect zeroing and calibration of monitor	Zero and calibrate monitor properly.	Recheck zero and calibration of monitor.
Loose connection	Use Luer-Lok stopcocks.	Check all connections.
	Use Luer-Lok stopcocks.	
Abnormally high pressure reading		
Pressure trapped by improper sequence of stopcock operation	Turn stopcocks in proper sequence when two pressures are measured on one transducer.	Thoroughly flush transducers with IV solution; rezero and turn stopcocks in proper sequence.
Incorrect air-reference level (below midchest level)	Maintain transducer air-reference port at midchest level; recheck and rezero after patient position changes.	Check air-reference level; reset at midchest and rezero.
Inappropriate pressure waveform		
Migration of catheter tip (e.g., in RV or PAW instead of in PA)	Establish optimal position carefully when introducing catheter initially.	Review waveform; if RV, inflate balloon; if PAW, deflate balloon and withdraw catheter slightly. Check position under fluoroscope and/or x-ray after reposition.
	Suture catheter at insertion site and tape catheter to patient's skin.	

3.32 ► Inaccurate Pulmonary Artery (PA) Pressure Measurements* *(continued)*

Problem/Cause	Prevention	Treatment
No pressure available		
Transducer not open to catheter	Follow routine, systematic steps for pressure measurement.	Check system, stopcocks.
Amplifiers still on cal, zero, or off		
Noise or fling in pressure waveform		
Excessive catheter movement, particularly in PA	Avoid excessive catheter length in ventricle.	Try different catheter tip position.
Excessive tubing length	Use shortest tubing possible (<3 to 4 feet).	Eliminate excess tubing.
Excessive stopcocks	Minimize number of stopcocks.	Eliminate excess stopcocks.

3.33 ▶ Troubleshooting Problems with Thermodilution Cardiac Output Measurements*

Problem	Cause	Action
Cardiac output values lower than expected	Injectate volume greater than designated amount	Inject exact volume to correspond to computation constant used.
		Discontinue rapid infusion through proximal or distal port.
	Catheter tip in RV or RA	Verify PA waveform from distal lumen. Reposition catheter.
	Incorrect computation constant (CC)	Reset computation constant. Correct prior CO values:
		Incorrect CO value $\times \dfrac{\text{correct CC}}{\text{wrong CC}}$
	Left-to-right shunt (VSD)	Check RA and PA oxygen saturations.
		Use alternative CO measurement technique.
	Catheter kinked or thermistor partially obstructed with clot	Check for kinks at insertion site; straighten catheter;
	Faulty catheter (communication between proximal and distal lumens)	aspirate and flush catheter. Replace catheter.

*RV, right ventricle; RA, right atrium; CO, cardiac output; VSD, ventricular septal defect; PA, pulmonary artery; PAW, pulmonary artery wedge; a-vDo$_2$, arteriovenous oxygen content difference; PVC, premature ventricular contraction; AF, atrial fibrillation.

From: Daily E, Schroeder J: Techniques in bedside hemodynamic monitoring, 5th ed. St. Louis, MO: CV Mosby, 1994, pp. 183–184. Cardiac output waveforms from: Gardner P: Cardiac output: Theory, technique and troubleshooting. In Underhill SL, Woods S, Froelicher E, et al: Cardiac nursing, 2nd ed. Philadelphia: JB Lippincott, 1989, p. 465.

3.33 ▶ Troubleshooting Problems with Thermodilution Cardiac Output Measurements* *(continued)*

Problem	Cause	Action
Cardiac output values higher than expected	Injectate volume less than designated amount	Inject exact volume to correspond to computation constant.
		Carefully remove all air bubbles from syringe.
	Catheter too distal (PAW)	Verify PA waveform from distal lumen.
		Pull catheter back.
	RA port lies within sheath	Advance catheter.
	Thermistor against wall of PA	Reposition patient.
		Rotate catheter to turn thermistor away from wall.
		Reposition catheter.
	Fibrin covering thermistor	Check a-vDo$_2$; change catheter.
	Incorrect computation constant (CC)	Correct prior CO values (see formula above).
		Reset computation constant.
	Right-to-left shunt (VSD)	Use alternative CO measurement technique.
	Severe tricuspid regurgitation	
	Incorrect injectate temperature	Use closed injectate system with in-line temperature probe.
		Handle syringe minimally.
		Do not turn stopcock to reestablish IV infusion through proximal port between injections; reduce or discontinue IV flow through VIP port.
		Try to determine cause or interference.

Problem	Cause	Action
Irregular upslope of CO curve	Magnetic interference producing numerous spikes in CO curve	Wipe CO computer with damp cloth.
	Long lag time between injection and upstroke of curve	Press start button after injection completed to delay computer sampling time.
	Uneven injection technique	Inject smoothly and quickly (10 ml in ≤ 4 seconds).
	RA port partially occluded with clot	Always check catheter patency by withdrawing, then flushing proximal port before CO determinations.
	Catheter partially kinked	Check for kinks, particularly at insertion site; straighten catheter; reposition patient.
	Cardiac dysrhythmias (PVC, AF, etc.)	Note ECG during CO determinations. Try to inject during a stable period. Increase the number of CO determinations.

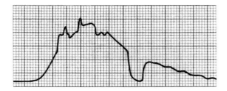

3.33 ▶ Troubleshooting Problems with Thermodilution Cardiac Output Measurements* *(continued)*

Problem	Cause	Action
Irregular downslope of CO curve	Marked movement of catheter tip	Obtain x-ray film to determine position of tip.
		Advance catheter tip away from pulmonic valve.
	Marked variation in PA baseline temperature	Use iced temperature injectate to increase signal/noise ratio.
		Increase the number of CO determinations.
		Inject at various times during respiratory cycle.
	Curve prematurely terminated	Press start button after injection completed to delay computer sampling time.
	Right-to-left shunt	Use alternative CO measurement technique.

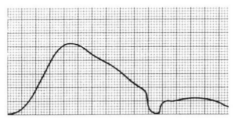

Respiratory System

4.1 ► Normal Chest X-Ray

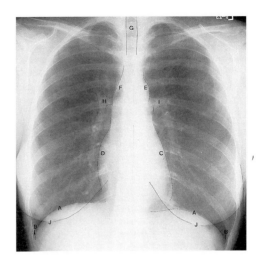

Normal chest x-ray film taken of a 28-year-old female from a posteroanterior (PA) view. The backward L in the upper right corner is placed on the film to indicate the left side of the chest. Some anatomic structures can be seen on the x-ray: (A) diaphragm; (B) costophrenic angle; (C) left ventricle; (D) right atrium; (E) aortic arch (referred to as aortic knob); (F) superior vena cava; (G) trachea; (H) right bronchus (right hilum); (I) left bronchus (left hilum); and (J) breast shadows.

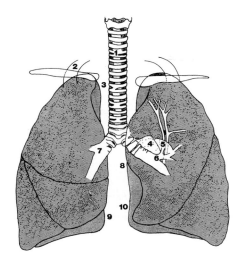

(1) Trachea, (2) first rib, (3) superior vena cava, (4) aortic knob, (5) pulmonary artery, (6) left main bronchus, (7) right main bronchus, (8) left atrium, (9) right atrium, and (10) left ventricle. *(From: Sanchez F: Fundamentals of chest x-ray interpretation.* Critical Care Nurse. *1986;6(5):53.)*

4.3 ▸ Acid-Base Abnormalities

Acid-Base Abnormality	Primary ABG Abnormalities			ABG Changes with Compensation (if present)	
	pH	Paco$_2$	HCO$_3^-$	Respiratory (Paco$_2$)	Metabolic (HCO$_3^-$)
Alkalemia					
Metabolic	↑		↑	↑	
Respiratory	↑	↓			↓
Acidemia					
Metabolic	↓		↓	↓	
Respiratory	↓	↑			↑

4.4 ▸ Indications for Mechanical Ventilation

Basic Physiologic Impairment	Best Available Indicators	Approximate Normal Range	Values Indicating Need for Ventilatory Support
Inadequate alveolar ventilation (acute ventilatory failure)	$Paco_2$, mm Hg	36–44	Acute increase from normal or patient's baseline
	Arterial pH	7.36–7.44	<7.25–7.30
Hypoxemia (acute oxygenation failure)	Alveolar-to-arterial Po_2 gradient breathing 100% O_2, mm Hg	25–65	>350
	Intrapulmonary right-to-left shunt fraction, percentage	<5	>20–25
	Pao_2/Fio_2, mm Hg	350–400	<200
Inadequate lung expansion	Tidal volume, ml/kg	5–8	<4–5
	Vital capacity	60–75	<10
	Respiratory rate, breaths/minute (adults)	12–20	>35
Inadequate respiratory muscle strength	Maximum inspiratory force, cm H_2O	−80–−100	<−25
	Maximum voluntary ventilation, L/minute	120–180	<2 × resting ventilatory requirement
	Vital capacity, ml/kg	60–75	<10–15

From: Luce J, Pierson D (eds.): Critical care medicine. *Philadelphia: WB Saunders, 1988, p. 219.*

4.4 ▶ Indications for Mechanical Ventilation *(continued)*

Basic Physiologic Impairment	Best Available Indicators	Approximate Normal Range	Values Indicating Need for Ventilatory Support
Excessive work of breathing	Minute ventilation necessary to maintain normal Pa_{CO_2}, L/minute	5–10	>15–20
	Dead space ratio, percentage	0.25–0.40	>0.60
	Respiratory rate, breaths/minute (adults)	12–20	>35
Unstable ventilatory drive	Breathing pattern; clinical setting		

4.5 ► Traditional Wean Criteria (Pulmonary Specific)

*Negative inspiratory pressure (NIP) ≤ -20 cm H_2O

Positive expiratory pressure (PEP) $\geq +30$ cm H_2O

*Spontaneous tidal volume (STV) ≥ 5 ml/kg

Vital capacity (VC) ≥ 10 to 15 ml/kg

*Fraction of inspired oxygen (Fio_2) $\leq 50\%$

*Minute ventilation (MV) ≤ 10 L/minute

*These criteria are considered the most reliable because they are not effort dependent.

4.6 ▶ Burns' Wean Assessment Program (BWAP)

Patient Name _____ Patient History

I. General Assessment

Yes	No	Not Assessed	
____	____	____	1. Hemodynamically stable (pulse rate, cardiac output)?
____	____	____	2. Free from factors that increase or decrease metabolic rate (seizures, temperature, sepsis, bacteremia, hypo/hyperthyroid)?
____	____	____	3. Hematocrit > 25% (or baseline)?
____	____	____	4. Systemically hydrated (weight at or near baseline, balanced intake and output)?
____	____	____	5. Nourished (albumin > 2.5, parenteral/enteral feedings maximized)? If albumin is low and anasarca or third spacing is present, score for hydration should be "no."
____	____	____	6. Electrolytes within normal limits (including Ca^{++}, Mg^+, PO_4)? Correct Ca^{++} for albumin level.
____	____	____	7. Pain controlled (subjective determination)?
____	____	____	8. Adequate sleep/rest (subjective determination)?
____	____	____	9. Appropriate level of anxiety and nervousness (subjective determination)?
____	____	____	10. Absence of bowel problems (diarrhea, constipation, ileus)?
____	____	____	11. Improved general body strength/endurance (i.e., out of bed in chair, progressive activity program)?
____	____	____	12. Chest x-ray improving?

II. Respiratory Assessment

Yes   No   Not Assessed

Gas Flow and Work of Breathing

——— ——— ———   13. Eupnic respiratory rate and pattern (spontaneous RR < 25, without dyspnea, absence of accessory muscle use)? This is assessed *off* the ventilator while measuring #20–23.

——— ——— ———   14. Absence of adventitious breath sounds (rhonchi, rales, wheezing)?

——— ——— ———   15. Secretions thin and minimal?

——— ——— ———   16. Absence of neuromuscular disease/deformity?

——— ——— ———   17. Absence of abdominal distention/obesity/ascites?

——— ——— ———   18. Oral ETT > #7.5 or trach > #7.5?

Airway Clearance

——— ——— ———   19. Cough and swallow reflexes adequate?

Strength

——— ——— ———   20. NIP < −20 (negative inspiratory pressure)?

——— ——— ———   21. PEP > +30 (positive expiratory pressure)?

Endurance

——— ——— ———   22. STV > 5 ml/kg (spontaneous tidal volume)?

——— ——— ———   23. VC > 10–15 ml/kg (vital capacity)?

ABG's

——— ——— ———   24. pH 7.30–7.45?

——— ——— ———   25. $PaCo_2 \sim 40$ mm Hg (or baseline) with MV <10 L/minute? This is evaluated while on ventilator.

——— ——— ———   26. $Pao_2 > 60$ on $Fio_2 < 40\%$?

4.7 ▸ Algorithm for Managing Ventilator Alarms and/or Acute Respiratory Distress

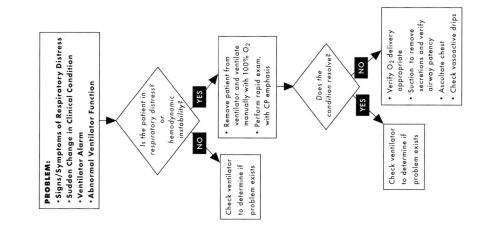

PROBLEM:
- **Signs/Symptoms of Respiratory Distress**
- **Sudden Change in Clinical Condition**
- **Ventilator Alarm**
- **Abnormal Ventilator Function**

Is the patient in respiratory distress? or hemodynamic instability?

YES — Remove patient from ventilator and ventilate manually with 100% O₂
- Perform rapid exam, with CP emphasis

NO — Check ventilator to determine if problem exists

Does the condition resolve?

YES — Check ventilator to determine if problem exists

NO — Verify O₂ delivery appropriate
- Suction to remove secretions and verify airway patency
- Auscultate chest
- Check vasoactive drips

4.8 ► Ventilatory Troubleshooting Guide

Problem/Causes	Management
Low exhaled tidal volume (TV)	
	Ventilate patient as necessary with manual resuscitation bag if exhibiting signs and symptoms of respiratory insufficiency and problem cannot be immediately corrected. Obtain appropriate assistance.
Patient-related: Cuff leak caused by:	Evaluate for cause of leak. Inflate cuff properly to minimally occlude trachea and provide effective ventilation.
• Insufficient air added to cuff	• If leak is in cuff, call for assistance in reintubation. Attempt to maintain ventilation in the interim by increasing TV to compensate for gas escaping or try leaving patient on ventilator and sealing mouth and nose with hands.
• Higher airway pressures, which create the need for higher cuff pressures to seal the trachea	Inform and reassure patient.
• Hole in cuff	Observe for potential gastric distension caused by leakage of air into stomach. Maintain gastric suction.
• Leak in air inflation port	• If leak is in air inflation port, seal port by placing three-way stopcock or leaving syringe on port. Tape syringe hub to prevent cuff deflation.
• Displaced endotracheal tube	• If endotracheal tube is displaced, reposition or obtain assistance as necessary.

Adapted from: Grossbach I: Trouble shooting ventilator and patient-related problems/parts I and II. Critical Care Nurse. 1989;6(4&5):58–70, 64–78.

4.8 ▶ Ventilatory Troubleshooting Guide *(continued)*

Problem/Causes	Management
Factors that increase airway resistance and/or decrease compliance (see Increased Airway Pressure) will increase inspiratory pressures and set off the high airway pressure alarm, causing the volume which is not delivered to be dumped from the ventilator. (Volume-cycled ventilators deliver the prescribed volume unless the pressure limit is exceeded.)	• Assess and correct causes of increased airway pressure (see Increased Airway Pressure). Increase airway pressure upper limit as necessary to allow for air delivery (last step after other assessments and management).
Bronchopleural air leak, which results in passage of air from airways to pleural space.	• Refer to Respiratory Acidosis section for management.
Ventilator-Related:	
Loose, cracked, ill-fitted connectors or humidifier.	• Check for loose, cracked, or ill-fitted humidity jar. Realign jar and tighten as necessary. Replace cracked jar.
Loose tubing, connections.	• Check for and tighten loose tubing connections.
Tears in tubing.	• Change tubing as necessary.
Flow rate may become too high because of a combination of high ventilator TV, rate, or flow rate settings. High flow rates may result in an inability to deliver the total prescribed volume.	• Be aware of potential volume loss resulting from combinations of high ventilator TV, respiratory rate, or peak flow settings, which exceed capabilities of the ventilator. (The effect of higher flow rates on volume delivery should be evaluated for the particular ventilator.) Correct problem by lowering the flow rate (decrease peak flow or lengthen inspiratory time; lower dialed-in respiratory rate or volume settings).
	• Support patient with manual resuscitation bag if unable to correct problem within 10 to 15 seconds. Call for assistance to change ventilators.

Problem/Causes	Management
No exhaled TV **Patient-related:** Patient disconnected from ventilator. Large cuff leak; endotracheal tube displaced so that cuff is above the vocal cords (may lead to inability to seal the pharyngeal area despite addition of large volume of air to cuff).	• Check patient to ensure that adaptor is attached to tracheostomy or endotracheal tube. • Evaluate and correct cuff leaks, endotracheal tube displacement.
Ventilator-related: Tubing disconnections, large tears in tubing, dislodged temperature sensing bag; loss of wall electrical or compressed air source.	• Evaluate for disconnected tubing, holes in tubing, loss of power or air/oxygen source.
Increased airway pressure **Patient-related:** Higher airway pressures are required to deliver the prescribed volume because of various factors that increase airway resistance, including secretions, mucous plugs, endotracheal tube factors (becomes kinked or narrowed, biting on orally placed tube), bronchospasm or decreased lung compliance, including pneumothorax, atelectasis, pulmonary edema. The upper airway pressure alarm sounds when the peak inspiratory pressure reaches the alarm limit which is set.	• Suction as necessary. • Assess for difficulty passing suction catheter through tube or observable kinking. Notify physician as necessary. • If patient bites on tube, explain purpose of tube, reason for not biting. • Anchor tube using tape or commercially designed tube holder if necessary. • Auscultate chest regularly to detect changes in breath sounds that may coincide with increased inspiratory pressures.

139

4.8 ▶ Ventilatory Troubleshooting Guide *(continued)*

Problem/Causes	Management
Endotracheal tube in right mainstem bronchus.	• Notify physician of decreased breath sounds. Obtain chest x-ray film to evaluate for proper endotracheal tube placement. Mark tube depth and anchor tube securely.
Inspiratory pressures can become higher because of resistance of the chest wall to expansion, abdominal pressure against the diaphragm, chest-wall injury, external restrictions, abdominal contractions during coughing or breathing efforts.	• Reposition patient for optimal ventilation. Increase upper pressure limit dial 10 to 15 cm H_2O higher than the pressure required for ventilation when certain positions that create higher pressures are necessary for patient management.
Coughing because of tracheal irritation caused by jarring of the endotracheal or tracheostomy tube; air leak around cuff, which causes air and secretion movement; head movement; tip of tube touching carina.	• Evaluate for causes of coughing (minimal or no volume delivery may occur if the high airway pressure alarm sounds because, when the set pressure limit is reached, inspiration is discontinued and expiration begins).
	• Avoid jarring or moving tube during turning.
	• Evaluate for optimum cuff inflation. Add air to cuff as necessary to "just seal" the trachea from air leakage that irritates airway and causes cough.
	• Chest x-ray studies to evaluate for proper tube placement.
	• Evaluate with physician whether patient is a candidate for weaning/ extubation, which will resolve the problem.
Need for communication of concerns and problems; may not be sufficiently informed or comprehending explanations regarding inability to verbally communicate; alternative methods of communication are not used or are inappropriate or ineffective.	• Explain reason for inability to communicate verbally and implement alternative method(s) to meet needs. Anticipate needs, ask "yes or no" questions.
	• Convey calm, confident, reassuring approach; explain procedures.

Problem/Causes	Management
Increased respiratory rate from anxiety, fear, pain, inadequate oxygenation, inadequate ventilation (hypercarbia), acidemia, or central nervous system malfunction. The higher the breathing rate, the faster the flow rates. If the ventilator peak flow rate is set too low or inspiratory time is too long, the patient will be attempting to exhale during the ventilator inspiratory phase. Forceful contraction of the thoracoabdominal musculature during the inspiratory phase causes the ventilator pressure limit to be exceeded, thus terminating air delivery prematurely.	• Evaluate for causes of increased ventilatory requirements, patient "fighting the ventilator" or "out of phase." Implement measures to correct problem(s). Provide calm, confident, reassuring approach. Explain interventions and use touch to relieve anxiety and fear. Provide analgesics as appropriate. Evaluate for increased work of breathing caused by inadequate oxygenation or ventilation caused by air leaks in the ventilator system. • Evaluate whether inspiratory flow rate setting is set optimally to match patient's breathing pattern. Observe chest/abdomen during inspiratory phase and evaluate whether patient appears to exhale (as evidenced by chest/abdominal contraction) during ventilator inspiratory cycle. Readjust peak flow dial higher or shorten inspiratory time and/or increase respiratory rate setting (higher setting results in increased flow rate) as necessary to match fast patient's inspiratory phase. • Observe trends in airway pressures which may signal changes in compliance. • If patient has status asthmaticus, provide sedation with morphine sulphate; pharmacologically paralyze as ordered to ensure optimal chest-wall compliance (decreases respiratory muscle activity and peak inspiratory pressures) and provide for adequate ventilation. Maintain on full ventilator support to minimize energy expenditure and maintain normal carbon dioxide levels. Provide bronchodilators, steroids, antibiotics as ordered.

4.8 ► Ventilatory Troubleshooting Guide *(continued)*

Problem/Causes	Management
Ventilator-related:	
Airway upper pressure limit alarm is set too low.	• Set upper pressure limit 10 to 15 cm H_2O higher than the patient's maximum inspiratory pressure.
Unusually high TV for the patient.	• Evaluate whether the patient is receiving too much TV (normal: 10 to 15 ml/kg normal body weight; 10 ml/kg in chronic lung disease).
	• Increase upper pressure limit.
	• Monitor for adverse effects of PEEP (see Decreased CO).
Compliance may be decreased when PEEP is applied, probably as a result of overdistension of alveoli.	• Increase upper pressure limit.
	• Monitor for adverse effects of PEEP (see Decreased CO).
Respiratory alkalosis	
Patient-Related:	
Factors that may increase respiratory rate or ventilation, including anxiety, restlessness, discomfort, pain; hypoxemia; central nervous system malfunction; metabolic acidosis; sensation of dyspnea caused by underlying lung pathology.	• Assist in decreasing feelings of anxiety and fear through calm, confident, reassuring approach, providing explanations and other measures to decrease stress.
	• Evaluate ventilator for proper functioning (receiving prescribed TV flow rate adjusted to match breathing pattern).
	• Check Pao_2, provide adequate oxygenation.
	• Evaluate and treat metabolic disturbance when warranted.
	• Consider different ventilation mode.
	• Consider that hyperventilation may not be corrected by various interventions because of central nervous system malfunction. Allow state of respiratory alkalosis.

Problem/Causes	Management
Mechanical hyperventilation ($Paco_2$ less than 28 mm Hg) may be used as therapy to decrease intracranial pressure.	• Mechanically hyperventilate as prescribed for purpose of decreasing intracranial pressure.
Ventilator-related: High tidal or minute volume settings on ventilator which cause overventilation, decreased $Paco_2$, increased pH.	• Set initial TV at 10 to 15 ml/kg and set rate at 8 to 12 breaths/minute. If patient has chronic obstructive pulmonary disease, select TV of about 10 ml/kg to reduce the risk of barotrauma and hyperventilation. Check arterial blood gases in about 20 minutes. • Decrease TV or respiratory rate if high. (NOTE: Decreasing respiratory rate setting while on assist/control mode will not correct the problem if the patient is triggering the ventilator. Decreasing TV may not correct the problem in patients who can maintain their desired $Paco_2$ level by increasing their respiratory rate.)
Too frequent or too many sighs. Machine sensitivity dial is set on positive side (versus negative 2 cm H_2O) causing machine to automatically cycle without patient effort, resulting in hyperventilation ($Paco_2$ below normal).	• Eliminate or decrease sighs. • Maintain sensitivity setting so that it takes -2 cm H_2O effort before a ventilator cycle can be initiated. • If patient is on PEEP, readjust sensitivity dial so that it is -2 to -3 cm H_2O less than the set PEEP value (e.g., for PEEP 5 cm H_2O, set sensitivity dial at $+ 2$ or 3 cm H_2O). NOTE: Some ventilators automatically reset sensitivity value when PEEP is applied. • When patient is on PEEP therapy, avoid air leaks in cuff or ventilator system (air leaks may cause loss of PEEP value and machine self-cycling occurs because sensitivity is set at a positive value).

4.8 ▸ Ventilatory Troubleshooting Guide *(continued)*

Problem/Causes	Management
Sensitivity needle (airway pressure needle) becomes maladjusted so that it rests at -2 cm H_2O level rather than resting at zero point, causing machine to self-cycle.	• Prior to placing patient on ventilator and prn, check ventilator sensitivity needle (airway pressure needle) to make sure it rests at zero point on airway pressure meter. Call respiratory therapist to readjust needle back to the zero point. Maintain 2 cm H_2O negativity with airway pressure needle. If ventilator does not have sensitivity dial with specific markings, regulate sensitivity setting by observing airway pressure needle. Regulate sensitivity dial so that the airway pressure needle registers 2 cm negativity with patient inspiratory effort.
Respiratory acidosis **Patient-related:** Inadequate TV to provide adequate gas exchange. Insufficient respiratory rate. Some COPD patients have chronically elevated $Paco_2$ levels.	• Increase TV. • Maintain $Paco_2$ at the patient's normal baseline level. Do not attempt to overventilate to a normal $Paco_2$ level if the patient has COPD with chronic carbon dioxide retention. • Make changes gradually to patient's baseline $Paco_2$ and pH. (Rapid changes may cause respiratory alkalosis with risk of cardiac arrhythmias, tetany, seizures.)

Problem/Causes	Management
Increased carbon dioxide production from the use of total parenteral nutrition (TPN) regimens containing high glucose loads. When carbohydrate (glucose) calories in TPN exceed a patient's metabolic demands, the surplus glucose is converted to fat through biochemical process associated with increased carbon dioxide production with small increase in oxygen consumption. Increased ventilation is observed as a result of increased carbon dioxide production. In mechanically ventilated patients unable to increase their minute ventilation (e.g., patients with chronic lung disease, those with normal lungs who develop compromised lung function because of acute lung disorder), the increase in carbon dioxide production is paralleled by an increase in $Paco_2$. Low ventilation to perfusion ratio of alveoli because of increased airway resistance or decreased compliance problems.	• Monitor effects of nutrition therapy on respiration, including measurements of minute ventilation, respiratory rate, oxygen consumption, carbon dioxide production, arterial blood gases. If increases in ventilation or carbon dioxide, or both, are noted after TPN has begun, the amount and source of nonprotein calories should be evaluated. • Particularly observe for TPN-induced acidosis in patients with chronic lung disease or marginal ventilatory reserve, who are on partial ventilator support (for example, IMV, CPAP, pressure support). • Discuss observations with physician so that changes can be made to limit glucose infusion and substitute fats for a portion of energy.

4.8 ▶ Ventilatory Troubleshooting Guide *(continued)*

Problem/Causes	Management
Bronchopleural air leak results in passage of air from airways to pleural space. Increased leak may occur because of factors tending to increase peak airway pressure during inspiration, such as high peak flow rate and high airway resistance. Increased mean intrathoracic pressure throughout the respiratory cycle, as occurs with a long inspiratory phase, inflation hold, expiratory retard, PEEP, and CPAP, will increase leak throughout the breath. Higher negative suction pressure will augment leak independent of factors as outlined here.	• Implement measures that minimize the bronchopleural pressure gradient, maintain adequate oxygenation and ventilation (pH greater than 7.30), keep lungs expanded, and control underlying disease process. Suggested conservative management includes: —Deliver lowest number of mechanical breaths compatible with adequate ventilation (spontaneous ventilation if possible). —Reduce exhaled TV to 10 ml/kg or less. —Adjust ventilator to minimize time spent in inspiration (short inspiratory time or high peak flow rate). —Avoid inflation hold and expiratory retard. —Avoid or minimize PEEP/CPAP. —Use lowest effective level of chest tube suction. —Explore positional differences on decreasing leak. —Sedate patient with or without paralysis if spontaneous movements accentuate leak. —Treat underlying cause for respiratory failure while maintaining nutritional and respiratory care support.

Problem/Causes	Management
Ventilator-related: Patient not receiving prescribed TV because of air leaks. Increased dead space on ventilator tubing. Reduction of volume delivered to the patient because of tubing system compliance and gas compression. This correction is generally in the range of 3 to 5 ml/cm H_2O of peak inspiratory pressure for adult ventilator circuits; however, may be negligible on some ventilator circuits.	• Evaluate and correct air leaks (refer to Low/No Exhaled TV sections. • Remove dead space tubing. • Be aware of reduced delivered volume, which may be significant if high inflation pressures are required. • Increase TV as necessary to provide adequate ventilation.

Thick secretions
  Patient-related:
    Dehydration.
 	
    Infection.
	• Maintain accurate intake, output, weight, CVP, LAP, PAWP recordings. Notify physician of abnormalities.
	• Maximize systemic hydration.
	• Monitor sputum for changes in color, amount, consistency. Obtain culture and sensitivity if indicated. If signs of infection, check with physician regarding antibiotics. Monitor for improvements after treatment initiated.
	• Suction as necessary if secretions present.

4.8 ► Ventilatory Troubleshooting Guide *(continued)*

Problem/Causes	Management
Ventilator-related: Heating unit set too low or not functioning properly. Insufficient water in humidifier jar.	• Check sensor that monitors temperature of inspired humidified gas (should be located close to patient airway). Maintain temperature at 98°F. • Notify respiratory therapist that heating unit not functioning properly. • Add water to refill line as necessary. Do not allow water to decrease below the refill line, which decreases effective humidification. • Drain water from tubing every 2 hours and prn.
Tracheostomy/endotracheal tube discomfort **Patient-related:** Insufficient attention to observing patient's airway, guiding tubing, and providing extra tubing during turning or other movement. Tube jarred with turning. Tube not secured adequately. Improvement in gas exchange because of improvement in disorder that caused increased oxygen requirement.	• Obtain necessary assistance so that one person can pay attention to guiding tubing and prevent pulling or jarring during patient activities. • Disconnect the patient from the ventilator, turn and reconnect. Do not leave off ventilator longer than 10 to 15 seconds. (Disconnection may be undesirable for patients requiring high oxygen concentrations, PEEP, or if they are paralyzed or sedated.) • Stabilize tracheostomy or endotracheal tube with one hand when reconnecting the ventilator adapter. • Anchor tube securely with ties or tape. • Position ventilator tubing on support system to minimize polling. • Recheck arterial blood gases in 15 to 20 minutes.

Problem/Causes	Management
Ventilator-related: Oxygen concentration setting on ventilator is too high.	• Decrease inspired oxygen concentration. • Recheck arterial blood gases in 15 to 20 minutes. • If on PEEP therapy, consider withdrawal of PEEP if Fio_2 less than 0.5. • Decrease PEEP in increments of 3 to 5 cm H_2O and evaluate arterial blood gases within 20 minutes. • Refer to Decreased CO section for other management procedures related to PEEP.
Low Pao_2/O_2 saturation **Patient-related:** Various abnormalities causing ventilation-perfusion disturbances and shunting, such as secretions, bronchospasm, pulmonary edema, pulmonary embolism. Arterial blood gas drawn immediately after suctioning. Changes in position causing alveolar hypoventilation, ventilation-perfusion disturbances. Right mainstem bronchus intubation, pneumothorax causing decreased ventilation.	• Correct pathophysiologic state causing the abnormal oxygenation. • Hyperoxygenate before and after suctioning as necessary (refer to Arrhythmias During Suctioning section). • Wait at least 15 to 20 minutes after suctioning before obtaining blood gas measurement. • Assess whether certain positions cause decreased Pao_2. Refrain from placing in positions which precipitate respiratory discomfort, unsafe drops in Pao_2, or obtain order to increase Fio_2 and/or TV for goals of maintaining adequate oxygenation, ventilation. • Evaluate for, and correct, tube malposition, pneumothorax. • Obtain chest x-ray film as necessary.

149

4.8 ► Ventilatory Troubleshooting Guide *(continued)*

Problem/Causes	Management
Ventilator-related: Oxygen concentration setting on ventilator is too low. Air leak around tracheostomy or endotracheal tube cuff, or in ventilator system, or both, leading to inadequate oxygenation, ventilation, loss of PEEP therapy. Inaccurate oxygen percentage from oxygen source failure or oxygen analyzer error.	• Increase Fio_2; add inspiratory pause, PEEP as necessary to avoid unsafe high oxygen concentrations. • Evaluate for air leaks, and correct (see Low/No Exhaled TV). • Notify respiratory therapist to determine accuracy of oxygen analyzer or whether oxygen concentration is being delivered. • Provide oxygen as necessary to maintain acceptable Pao_2.
Decreased cardiac output (CO) with hypotension **Patient-related:** Significant stimulation (hypoxemia, hypercarbia, acidemia) of the autonomic system in a patient requiring ventilator support. Physiologic stress is frequently compounded by a state of anxiety and fear. These factors lead to arterial and venous constriction, as well as myocardial stimulation. Support of ventilation usually relieves work of breathing, and reverses hypercarbia, acidemia, and hypoxemia. It also produces relaxation and sleep, and may induce unconsciousness. The combination of loss of consciousness, relief of breathing work, and improved oxygenation and ventilation often leads to a profound and sudden	• Be aware of potential hypotension following institution of positive pressure ventilation. Monitor blood pressure, pulse, rhythm. • Stabilize cardiovascular system by correcting relative hypovolemia with appropriate intravenous fluid administration. • Elevate lower extremities 20 to 30 degrees from horizontal position if hypotension is severe. • During this period, augment spontaneous ventilation initially by manual ventilation (using technique which maintains synchrony with the patient's varying inspiratory efforts and leads to a profound and sudden decrease in sympathetic stimulation to the cardiovascular system, which results in

Problem/Causes	Management

decrease in sympathetic stimulation to the cardiovascular system, which results in arteriolar and venous relaxation and a significant increase in the vascular space.

Sudden "relative hypovolemia" may occur because the patient cannot mobilize extravascular fluid rapidly. Positive ventilator pressure increases intrathoracic pressure and accentuates interference with venous return, making relative hypovolemia significant.

Intravascular volume depletion; when PEEP therapy produces significant reductions in cardiac output despite intravascular volume augmentation, an element of ventricular dysfunction may be involved.

arteriolar dilatation and allows the patient to "fight" the positive pressure, which increases intrathoracic pressure.

- Make sure the manual ventilation bag is capable of providing adequate oxygenation and ventilation to meet the patient's requirements.
- Place patient on ventilator when relaxed. Shorten inspiratory time or increase peak flow dial as necessary to simulate normal breathing pattern.
- Monitor vital signs, hemodynamic parameters, if pulmonary artery catheter in place, including: (1) arterial venous oxygen content difference and CO measurements (aids assessment of perfusion and oxygen extraction); (2) intrapulmonary shunt calculations (aids assessment of pulmonary effects of PEEP); and (3) pulmonary artery occlusion pressures (aids in the assesment of intravascular fluid administration). Notify physician of abnormalities.
- Administer IV fluids to correct intravascular hypovolemia.

4.8 ▶ Ventilatory Troubleshooting Guide *(continued)*

Problem/Causes	Management
Patients with airflow obstruction may trap air so that alveolar pressure remains positive at end-expiration, even when PEEP is not applied intentionally. This "auto-PEEP" effect can cause increased intrathoracic pressure and severely depress CO. It is likely to develop if gas exchange is prolonged by increases in thoracic compliance or resistance, or if the time for exhalation is shortened by a high ventilatory requirement. Auto-PEEP can develop whenever the minute ventilation is great enough that the lung cannot empty to its usual relaxed volume between inflations. The magnitude of intrinsic PEEP increases with decreased duration of expiration.	• Evaluate auto-PEEP in patients with airflow obstruction (performed by occluding expiratory port at end-expiration by the ventilator or pressing end-expiration hold button on some ventilators) and observe positive pressure registered on airway-pressure manometer. No spontaneous respiratory efforts should be present nor any gas flow from a supplemental source, such as that used in some IMV systems or medication nebulization. • Treat hemodynamic effects of auto-PEEP by measures that lower mean intrathoracic pressure. 　—Adjust inspiratory time or peak flow setting to allow maximal time for exhalation between cycles (shorten inspiratory time or increase peak flow) and to avoid progressive increases in end-expiratory lung volume, hyperinflation. 　—Reduce minute ventilation to minimal amount consistent with acceptable pH. 　—Try higher TV (not usually effective if minute ventilation remains unchanged) or IMV. 　—Correct fever, agitation, metabolic acidosis, to diminish ventilatory requirements. 　—Continue medical therapy for treatment of airflow obstruction. • Administer fluids to correct hypovolemia.

Problem/Causes	Management
	• Administer inotropic agents as necessary. • Increase PEEP in increments of 3 to 5 cm H_2O. Monitor for signs, symptoms of decreased CO. Evaluate arterial blood gases within 20 to 30 minutes of setting change.
Level of PEEP is unnecessarily high for therapeutic goal of adequate arterial oxygen content without significant reduction in CO at FiO_2 below 0.5. Oxygen concentrations greater than 0.5 over prolonged periods can result in oxygen toxicity.	• Use the lowest level of PEEP necessary to correct severe hypoxemia (result PaO_2 greater than 60 mm Hg under most circumstances) while allowing a reduction of the FiO_2 below 0.5. • Provide PEEP if an FiO_2 of greater than 0.5 is required for more than 24 hours to achieve a PaO_2 greater than 50 to 60 mm Hg. NOTE: "Enough" PEEP has been applied when, in the presence of adequate perfusion and hemoglobin content, a PaO_2 of at least 60 mm Hg is achieved at an FiO_2 of 0.4 or less.
Ventilator-Related: Positive pressure ventilation and PEEP may decrease CO by impeding venous return, which decreases right and subsequently left ventricular stroke volume. Other factors proposed may include release of humoral substances during lung expansion, which depress left ventricular function and CO reduction secondary to endocardial blood supply impairment. Factors that may increase positive intrathoracic pressure and mean airway pressure include high TV, PEEP, continuous mechanical ventilation, and increased respiratory rate (more positive pressure).	• May need to decrease TV to avoid high peak inspiratory pressures. • Use TV and PEEP that maintain "optimal compliance." • Avoid use of inspiratory pause or hold. • May try shortening inspiratory time or increasing peak flow to shorten the amount of time that positive pressure remains in the thorax and prevent "fighting" of positive pressure, which unduly increases intrathoracic pressure. • Use lowest PEEP level necessary to meet therapeutic goal. • Increase FiO_2 and remove PEEP as necessary until the patient is hemodynamically stabilized.

4.8 ▶ Ventilatory Troubleshooting Guide *(continued)*

Problem/Causes	Management
A higher intrapleural pressure and lower CO may be produced when PEEP is used on control mode and pressure ventilation versus PEEP with spontaneous ventilation (CPAP) or IMV.	• May try IMV or CPAP mode if compatible with cardiovascular and clinical stability to lower intrapleural pressures and reduce harmful alterations in cardiac function.

Anxiety and fear
  Patient-Related:
  Decreased ability to communicate because of tracheostomy/ endotracheal tube. Fear of unknown, unfamiliar environment and people.
	• Assess most effective method(s) of communication: paper and pencil, lip reading, gestures, alphabet board, cards indicating major needs, and electric larynx. Communicate method on care plan.
	• Ask "yes and no" questions.
	• Keep call light in reach at all times.
	• Obtain assistance if unable to interpret communications. Use touch to ease frustrations.
	• Evaluate and manage psychosocial factors that may be creating anxiety and fear.
	• Convey calm, confident, reassuring approach.
	• Explain all procedures, allow patient participation in decisions to the extent possible.
	• Maintain familiarity in environment (family visits, significant personal belongings, radio, television, clock, consistency in personnel caring for patient).

Problem/Causes	Management
Effects of surgery or various other interventions, which create discomfort, pain. Decreased arterial oxygenation related to suctioning.	• Identify factors creating discomfort, pain, shortness of breath, and implement measures to modify or resolve problem. • See Low Pao$_2$ and Arrhythmias During Suctioning.
Ventilator-Related: Ventilator settings not optimally adjusted to meet patient's needs. Air leaks causing patient to receive inadequate ventilation, oxygenation; incorrect settings.	• Assess whether ventilator is optimally adjusted to meet patient's needs. Readjust flow rate setting higher or inspiratory time shorter as necessary to match faster breathing pattern. • Evaluate whether prescribed TV is being delivered and whether settings are correct. Manually ventilate as necessary. • Efficiently identify and correct problem using a calm, confident approach.

4.8 ► Ventilatory Troubleshooting Guide *(continued)*

Problem/Causes	Management

Arrhythmias during or after suctioning
   Patient-Related:
   Suctioning induces arterial desaturation. Other adverse effects include bronchoconstriction, vasovagal reactions, cardiac arrhythmias, unexplained cardiovascular collapse and sudden death.

   There are considerable differences in the rate of fall in oxygen tension. Variables affecting the degree of hypoxemia include: (1) the ratio of suction catheter size to endotracheal tube size, (2) the duration of suctioning, (3) whether or not hyperoxygenation was performed before or after suctioning, (4) the patient's initial Pao_2, (5) the magnitude of pulmonary shunt, (6) suction-induced alveolar collapse, (8) the ability to breathe spontaneously.

• Implement measures to minimize or prevent suction-related hypoxemia and vagal reactions:
   —Assess need for suctioning. Suction only as necessary, not on a "routine" basis.
   —Use catheter no greater than half the diameter of the tube through which it is passed.
   —Inform patient that you will be suctioning.
   —Insert catheter without applying suction.
   —Spend less than 15 seconds total time off ventilator. Limit applied suction time to 10 seconds.
   —Administer hyperoxygenation (100% O_2) with a manual resuscitation bag or the ventilator for 3 to 5 breaths before and after each suctioning pass.
   —Use ventilator for hyperoxygenation when PEEP > 10 cm H_2O or when removal from ventilator results in distress or hypoxemia.
   —Monitor blood pressure, heart rate, rhythm during suctioning procedures. If arrhythmias or significant changes in heart rate occur, discontinue suctioning and ventilate patient immediately using 100% O_2 for several breaths. Be certain that vital signs have returned to baseline values before repeating suction process.

Problem/Causes	Management
	—Modify procedure for pre- and post-hyperoxygenation to fit the individual patient's psychologic requirements.
	• Assess whether an increase in Fio_2 or mechanical hyperinflation with oxygen is needed to raise the Pao_2 to a sufficient level. If mechanical hyperinflation is needed, avoid large changes in pH (respiratory alkalosis) which may produce hazards related to myocardial and central nervous system excitability.
Large lung volumes have been reported to cause bradycardia and hypotension.	• Stop hyperinflation if serious hypotension or bradycardia is observed.
	• Be knowledgeable about oxygen delivery performance of resuscitation bag or device used (oxygen delivery varies with differnt types). If the Fio_2 is increased on the ventilator, keep in mind that a variable lag time will elapse before the patient receives the increased oxygen concentration because of the "washout" time of the ventilator.
	• Keep patient on the ventilator during atrial pressure measurements.
	• Consider use of an adapter that allows the patient to remain on the ventilator during suctioning.
	NOTE: May produce smaller decreases in Pao_2 than does suctioning when the ventilator is removed. This method may be preferred if patient is unresponsive to increased oxygen concentrations because of large pulmonary shunts.

4.8 ► Ventilatory Troubleshooting Guide *(continued)*

Problem/Causes	Management
Ventilator performance during suctioning is a critical factor in determining whether suctioning through an adapter in a closed airway can be done safely. If suctioning is performed in a closed airway system and suction flow exceeds volume of gas supplied by the ventilator, negative airway pressure can reduce lung volume and cause alveolar collapse and arterial desaturation.	• Be alert to potential complications of hypoxemia during closed airway suctioning related to suction flow exceeding gas delivery by the ventilator. Discontinue method.
Receptors for the vagus nerve are found throughout the tracheobronchial tree, to the level of the carina. Stimulation of this nerve produces slowing of the heart rate.	• Monitor blood pressure and heart rate during suctioning procedure. Discontinue suctioning if significant decrease in blood pressure and heart rate occurs and ventilate patient.
Mechanical ventilation increases intrathoracic pressures to Valsalva levels. The increased intrathoracic pressure that occurs during Valsalva's maneuver (coughing, vomiting, lifting, the act of defecating) causes rapid changes in preload and afterload. During strain, venous return to the heart is decreased and systolic and pulse pressures decrease. Paroxysms of coughing without taking a deep breath are Valsalva strains at high expiratory pressures.	• Be alert to potential complications related to coughing against the obstruction of the suction catheter plus additional increased intrathoracic pressure if the closed airway system is in place. Monitor for slowing of heart rate, decreased blood pressure.
	• Remove the catheter from the trachea when the patient coughs.
	• If the closed airway suction system has been used, evaluate whether the problem is resolved by the method of removing patient from the ventilator and suctioning. Discontinue use of closed airway suction system.

Problem/Causes	Management
Incorrect PEEP setting 　**Patient-Related:** 　　Unable to accurately read airway pressure gauge for determining PEEP setting because of patient's fast respiratory rate, irregular respiratory pattern or imcomplete exhalations, or both.	• Adjust PEEP while the patient is on the ventilator unless difficulty arises in making accurate adjustments because of certain breathing patterns, which prevent accurate observation of the airway pressure needle. In this case, adjust PEEP by removing patient from ventilator, attaching test balloon to ventilator, and adjusting PEEP. Obtain assistance of second person to support patient by manual resuscitation bag. • Reset sensitivity setting so that it is 2 or 3 cm H_2O less than the dialed-in PEEP value (step not necessary on some ventilators where the sensitivity automatically readjusts when PEEP is applied).
Air leak in patient (cuff site) or ventilator system causing inability to maintain end-expiratory pressure. If air leak is corrected, the previously set PEEP value will register higher if PEEP was set while an air leak was present in the system.	• Evaluate and correct air leaks (see Low/No Exhaled Volume). • Recheck PEEP value after leak is corrected; readjust PEEP as necessary.

4.8 ► Ventilatory Troubleshooting Guide *(continued)*

Problem/Causes	Management
Ventilator-Related: PEEP incorrectly set on machine. Ventilator sensitivity setting is set so that the machine self-cycles; the airway pressure needle may rest at a positive value, which results in a false appearance of PEEP. If air leaks develop in the ventilator system or cuff, ventilator self-cycling occurs because of loss of PEEP with a machine sensitivity setting at a positive value.	• Assess whether PEEP is correctly set. Reset as necessary. • Set sensitivity dial so that it is 2 or 3 cm H_2O less than the dialed-in PEEP value. • Rule out the possibility of machine self-cycling by decreasing sensitivity temporarily to -2 cm H_2O (or significantly less than the PEEP setting, if on higher levels) and noting whether the respiratory rate decreases or the prescribed PEEP value registers on the airway pressure gauge. Correct air leaks. • Be suspicious of machine self-cycling if the patient does not appear to be generating muscle activity to assist or is obviously not assisting (effects of drugs) despite high respiratory rate. • Prevent air leaks, which may lead to loss of PEEP and machine self-cycling.
Pneumothorax/tension pneumothorax Defective PEEP value or regulator.	• Change PEEP valves. Notify respiratory therapist of problem maintaining desired PEEP level.
Patient-Related: Underlying lung pathology (COPD, emphysematous blebs, lung surgery), which makes some persons more susceptible to the effects of positive pressure.	

Problem/Causes	Management
Ventilator-Related: Positive pressure created by ventilator, which causes pulmonary barotrauma. High volume or high pressure settings, PEEP.	• Use PEEP only as necessary. • Maintain minimal PEEP levels necessary for adequate oxygenation. • Try ventilator modes with low mean airway pressure levels to decrease mean intrathoracic pressure. • Monitor for signs, symptoms of pneumothorax, tension pneumothorax. Notify physician of abnormalities. • If symptoms are mild, obtain chest x-ray film and notify physician immediately. • If tension pneumothorax occurs: —Disconnect patient from ventilator and ventilate with manual resuscitation bag. —Increase Fio_2 to 1.0. —Have someone else notify physician immediately, prepare chest tube insertion equipment for immediate use and set up chest drainage unit. —Have a large-bore needle ready for insertion as a life-saving maneuver for tension pneumothorax. NOTE: Needle thoracentesis is performed using a medium or large-bore needle, which is inserted into the affected hemithorax anteriorly through the second or third interspace in the midclavicular line. The needle should pass through the middle of the interspace to avoid intercostal blood vessels.

4.8 ▶ Ventilatory Troubleshooting Guide *(continued)*

Problem/Causes	Management
	• Reassure, remain with the patient. • Obtain chest x-ray film. • Monitor arterial blood gases every 1 to 2 hours until stable.

Inability to tolerate IMV mode
  Patient-Related:
  Increased work of breathing from various physiologic factors that increase airway resistance, decrease lung compliance, decrease respiratory muscle strength and endurance, or alter mechanics of breathing; includes:

  • Secretions, infection

  • Narrowed airway because of endotracheal tube. (Airway resistance has been reported to increase threefold and the work of breathing almost twofold by size 7- to 9-mm endotracheal tubes. Even a 9-mm tube increased work of breathing 77.6 percent above baseline.)

  • Bronchospasm.

Management column:

• Support on ventilator mode which provides patient comfort.

• Suction airway as necessary. Provide call light so that capable patient can inform of need.
• Provide medications as ordered for management of respiratory infection.
• Consider endotracheal tube diameter as one of the factors which may increase airway resistance and work of breathing.
• Change to different mode of ventilation or add pressure support if it provides breathing comfort.
• Use t-tube method for weaning from the ventilator when physiologically stable. Suggest extubation after a short t-tube trial (20 to 30 minutes) or some patients may not need t-tube trial.
• Evaluate, treat bronchospasm.

Problem/Causes	Management
• Certain positions which provide less than optimal ventilation-perfusion matching. • Acute or chronic lung disorder, or both. • Inadequate IMV rate or volume to maintain adequate ventilation for the patient under effects of narcotics and anesthetics. • Decreased respiratory muscle strength and endurance from effects of malnutrition. Increased carbon dioxide production resulting from the use of TPN regimens containing carbohydrate (glucose) concentrations. Increased respiratory rate and ventilation may be observed as a result of the increased carbon dioxide production. (See Respiratory Acidosis.)	• Place in positions that maximize ventilation and breathing comfort (usually with head of bed elevated). • Evaluate whether the patient is physiologically stable enough to be on partial ventilator support. • Provide necessary ventilator support for goals of breathing comfort, ability to rest and sleep, and maintain normal ventilation, oxygenation. May try increasing rate or volume, or both, if settings are low, otherwise switch to assist/control mode, particularly if patient is not tolerating IMV mode. • Observe for TPN-induced hypercapnic acidosis in patients with chronic lung disease or marginal ventilatory reserve who are on partial ventilatory support (for example, IMV, CPAP, pressure support). • Discuss observations with physician so that changes can be made to limit glucose infusion and substitute fats for a portion of energy. • Provide optimum ventilator support by placing on assist/control mode. • Support patient on the ventilatory mode, which provides respiratory comfort, usually assist/control mode. • Thoroughly assess and correct any physiologic and equipment factors interfering with success.

4.8 ▶ Ventilatory Troubleshooting Guide *(continued)*

Problem/Causes	Management
	• Wean only as tolerated using t-tube method. Abide by proper procedure, which includes suctioning as necessary, optimum positioning, close monitoring, and provision of a reassuring, confident, and consistent approach. Provide ventilator support as necessary to avoid physiologic decompensation and deterioration of patient trust and confidence.
Ventilator-Related: Various equipment factors can significantly increase resistance and work of breathing, which cause various signs and symptoms of respiratory distress. These include resistance in the IMV demand valve, or system, and in the ventilator breathing circuit. A significant increase in resistance results if the flow rate delivered by the IMV apparatus is lower than the patient's spontaneous inspiratory flow rate or if the demand valve requires significant airway pressure deflection to initiate air flow during spontaneous breathing. Resistance varies in the various ventilator breathing circuits. Persons with COPD are at high risk for development of inspiratory muscle fatigue which may precipitate acute respiratory failure. Weaning failures may be the result of improper use of the IMV method, which can unnecessarily prolong the length of time that patients spend on the ventilator. Delay of the weaning process and extubation may also occur due to gradual reduction in ventilatory rate.	• Become knowledgeable about the particular IMV system in use, including specific capabilities, limitations, correct setup, and usual problems. • If patient develops respiratory distress after placement on IMV mode, switch to assist/control mode (or previous mode of respiratory comfort). Notify respiratory therapist for problem identification and management.

Problem/Causes	Management
Deleterious effects on hemodynamic status may occur when patients with poor left ventricular reserve are changed from controlled mechanical ventilation to IMV. Oxygen consumption can increase significantly at lower IMV rate. Myocardial ischemia has been shown to occur more often on CPAP versus full ventilator support. Mechanical ventilator support may be beneficial to the failing heart in several ways: optimizes left ventricular end-diastolic volume (increases intrapleural pressure which decreases right heart preload; increased airway pressure may restrict left ventricular filling); in clinical states of compromised oxygen delivery (cardiogenic shock), full ventilatory support may decrease inspiratory oxygen demands and release oxygen for use by other systems; patients can be safely sedated and sympathetic outflow is decreased, which prevents hypertension and tachycardia thereby decreasing left ventricular strain. Kinked tubing, obstruction of tubing with water.	• Monitor for deleterious effects of partial ventilator support on hemodynamic status, particularly in some patients, such as those in cardiogenic shock, whose clinical status requires a low oxygen consumption. • In the presence of cardiogenic shock, provide optimum ventilator support to decrease inspiratory oxygen demands. • Drape tubing to avoid kinks and for optimum drainage of water into water traps. Empty water from tubing every 2 to 4 hours.

4.8 ▶ Ventilatory Troubleshooting Guide *(continued)*

Problem/Causes	Management
Setting incorrectly calculated, set on machine.	• Evaluate whether IMV settings are correctly dialed on ventilator. Correct errors or notify respiratory therapist as necessary.
Inappropriate inspiratory time or flow rate setting.	• Evaluate for appropriate inspiratory time or peak flow setting by observing speed of chest expansion on positive pressure breaths. (Rapid rise of the chest and airway pressure needle may be indicators that the inspiratory time is too short or peak flow too fast.) Notify respiratory therapist or make appropriate inspiratory time or peak flow adjustments.
Incorrect assembly of IMV setup, malfunctioning IMV valve which creates additional resistance.	• Switch to assist/control mode or settings that provide optimum ventilation, oxygenation, and breathing comfort or ventilate patient using manual resuscitation bag if unfamiliar with machine settings. Notify respiratory therapist for correction of problem.
Not receiving prescribed TV because of air leaks in ventilator system or cuff.	• Check whether machine is delivering prescribed positive pressure breaths by observing digital display on some ventilators or by switching to assist/control mode and evaluating volume delivery on other ventilators (see Low/No Exhaled TV).
Some IMV systems are not synchronized with the patient's inspiratory efforts (i.e., the machine breaths are initiated at any point during the respiratory cycle). Asynchrony may create feelings of discomfort and frustration, especially with higher IMV rates. Stacking of breaths may increase intrapleural pressure, cause overdistension of alveoli and barotrauma.	• Switch to assist/control mode as necessary. If ready for weaning, use t-tube method, extubate.

Pharmacology Tables

5.1 ► Intravenous Medication Administration Guidelines

Drug	Usual IV Dose Range*	Standard Dilution	Infusion Times/Comments/Drug Interactions
Acetazolamide	5 mg/kg/24h or 250 mg qd-qid	Undiluted	Infuse at 500 mg/minute
Acyclovir	5 mg/kg q8h	D5W 100 ml	Infuse over at least 60 minutes
Adenosine	6 mg initially, then 12 mg × 2 doses	Undiluted	Inject over 1–2 seconds Drug interactions; theophylline (1); persantine (2)
Amikacin			
Standard dose	7.5 mg/kg q12h	D5W 50 ml	Infuse over 30 minutes
Single daily dose	20 mg/kg q24h	D5W 50 ml	Drug interactions: neuromuscular blocking agents (3) Therapeutic levels: Peak: 20–40 mg/L; trough: <8 mg/L Single daily dose: trough level at 24 hours = 0 mg/L; peak levels unnecessary

*Usual dose ranges are listed; refer to appropriate disease state for specific dose.

Abbreviations: IVP, IV push; IVPB, IV piggy back; D5W, dextrose-5%-water; NS, normal saline; SW, sterile water.

Drug interactions: (1) antagonizes adenosine effect; (2) potentiates adenosine effect; (3) potentiates effect of neuromuscular blocking agents; (4) inhibits theophylline metabolism; (5) antagonizes effect of neuromuscular blocking agents; (6) metabolism inhibited by cimetidine; (7) metabolism inhibited by ciprofloxacin; (8) increased digoxin concentrations; (9) metabolism inhibited by erythromycin; (10) increased nephrotoxicity; (11) increased heparin requirements.

5.1 ► Intravenous Medication Administration Guidelines *(continued)*

Drug	Usual IV Dose Range*	Standard Dilution	Infusion Times/Comments/Drug Interactions
Aminophylline			
Loading dose	6 mg/kg	D5W 50 ml	Infuse loading dose over 30 minutes Maximum loading infusion rate 25 mg/minute Aminophylline = 80% theophylline Drug interactions: cimetidine, ciprofloxacin, erythromycin, clarithromycin (4)
Infusion dose		500 mg in D5W 500 ml	Therapeutic levels: 10–20 mg/L
CHF	0.3 mg/kg/hour		
Normal	0.6 mg/kg/hour		
Smoker	0.9 mg/kg/hour		
Ammonium chloride	mEq Cl = Cl deficit (in mEq/L × 0.2 × wt (kg)	100 mEq in NS 500 ml	Maximum infusion rate is 5 ml/minute of a 0.2-mEq/ml solution; correct 1/3 to 1/2 of Cl deficit while monitoring pH and Cl; administer remainder as needed
Amphotericin B	0.5–1.5 mg/kg q24h	D5W 250 ml	Infuse over 2–6 hours Do not mix in electrolyte solutions (e.g., saline, Ringer's lactate)
Ampicillin	0.5–3 g q4–6h	NS 100 ml	Infuse over 15–30 minutes
Ampicillin/sulbactam	1.5–3 g q6h	NS 100 ml	Infuse over 15–30 minutes

5.1 ▸ Intravenous Medication Administration Guidelines *(continued)*

Drug	Usual IV Dose Range*	Standard Dilution	Infusion Times / Comments / Drug Interactions
Amrinone			
Loading dose	0.75–3 mg/kg	Undiluted	Inject over 1–2 minutes Do not mix in dextrose-containing solutions; may be injected into running dextrose infusions through a Y-connector or directly into tubing
Infusion dose	5–20 μg/kg/minute	300 mg in NS 120 ml	
Anistreplase (APSAC)	30 U IV	SW 5 ml	Infuse over 5 minutes, give with aspirin 325 mg PO immediately Preparation should be discarded if not used within 6 hours
Atenolol	5 mg IV over 5 minutes, 5 mg IV 10 minutes later	Undiluted	Inject 1 mg/minute
Atracurium			
Intubating dose	0.4–0.5 mg/kg	Undiluted	Inject over 60 seconds to prevent histamine release
Maintenance dose	0.08–0.1 mg/kg	Undiluted	Inject over 60 seconds to prevent histamine release
Infusion dose	5–9 μg/kg/minute	1000 mg in D5W 150 ml	Continuous infusion. Final volume = 250 ml, conc = 4 mg/ml Drug interactions: aminoglycosides (3); anticonvulsants (5)
Aztreonam	0.5–2 g q6–12 h	D5W 100 ml	Infuse over 15–30 minutes
Bretylium			
Bolus dose	5–10 mg/kg	Undiluted	Infuse over 5–10 seconds
Infusion dose	1–5 mg/minute	2 g in D5W 500 ml	Continuous infusion

Drug	Usual IV Dose Range*	Standard Dilution	Infusion Times / Comments / Drug Interactions
Bumetanide			
Bolus dose	0.5–1 mg	Undiluted	Maximum injection rate: 1 mg/minute
Infusion dose	0.08–0.3 mg/hour	2.4 mg in NS 100 ml	Continuous infusion
Calcium (elemental)	100–200 mg of elemental calcium IV over 15 minutes followed by 100 mg/hour	1000 mg in NS 1000 ml	Ca chloride 1 g = 272 mg (13.6 mEq) of elemental calcium Ca gluconate 1 g = 90 mg (4.65 mEq) of elemental calcium
Cefamandole	0.5–2 g q4–8h	D5W 50 ml	Infuse over 15–30 minutes
Cefazolin	0.5–1 g q6–8h	D5W 50 ml	Infuse over 15–30 minutes
Cefmetazole	2 g q6–12h	D5W 50 ml	Infuse over 15–30 minutes
Cefonicid	1–2 g q24h	D5W 50 ml	Infuse over 15–30 minutes
Cefoperazone	1–2 g q12h	D5W 50 ml	Infuse over 15–30 minutes
Cefotaxime	1–2 g q4–6h	D5W 50 ml	Infuse over 15–30 minutes
Cefotetan	1–2 g q12h	D5W 50 ml	Infuse over 15–30 minutes
Cefoxitin	1–2 g q4–6h	D5W 50 ml	Infuse over 15–30 minutes
Ceftazidime	0.5–2 g q8–12h	D5W 50 ml	Infuse over 15–30 minutes
Ceftizoxime	1–2 g q8–12h	D5W 50 ml	Infuse over 15–30 minutes
Ceftriaxone	0.5–2 g q12–24h	D5W 50 ml	Infuse over 15–30 minutes
Cefuroxime	0.75–1.5 g q8h	D5W 50 ml	Infuse over 15–30 minutes
Chlorothiazide	0.5–1 g qd-bid	SW 18 ml	Inject over 3–5 minutes

5.1 ▶ Intravenous Medication Administration Guidelines *(continued)*

Drug	Usual IV Dose Range*	Standard Dilution	Infusion Times / Comments / Drug Interactions
Chlorpromazine	10–50 mg q4–6h	Dilute with NS to a final concentration of 1 mg/ml	Inject at 1 mg/minute
Cimetidine			
IVPB	300 mg q6–8h	D5W 50 ml	Infuse over 15–30 minutes IVP dose may be injected over at least 5 minutes
Infusion dose	37.5 mg/hour	D5W 250 ml	Continuous infusion Drug interactions: theophylline, warfarin, phenytoin, lidocaine, benzodiazepines (6)
Ciprofloxacin	200–400 mg q12h	Premix solution 2 mg/ml	Infuse over 60 minutes Drug interactions: theophylline, warfarin (7)
Clindamycin	150–900 mg q8h	D5W 100 ml	Infuse over 30–60 minutes
Conjugated estrogens	0.6 mg/kg/d × 5 days	NS 50 ml	Infuse over 15–30 minutes
Cosyntropin	0.25 mg IV	Undiluted	Inject over 60 seconds
Cyclosporine	5–6 mg/kg q24h	D5W 100 ml	Infuse over 2–6 hours Drug interactions: digoxin (8); erythromycin (9); amphotericin, NSAID (10) IV dose = 1/3 PO dose Therapeutic levels: trough: 50–150 ng/ml (whole blood-HPLC)

Drug	Usual IV Dose Range*	Standard Dilution	Infusion Times / Comments / Drug Interactions
Dantrolene			
Bolus dose	1–2 mg/kg	SW 60 ml	Administer as rapidly as possible
Maximum dose	10 mg/kg		Do not dilute in dextrose or electrolyte-containing solutions
Maintenance dose	2.5 mg/kg q4h × 24h	SW 60 ml	Infuse over 60 minutes
Desmopressin	0.3 mg/kg	NS 50 ml	Infuse over 15–30 minutes
Dexamethasone	0.5–20 mg	NS 50 ml	May give doses ≤ 10 mg undiluted IVP over 60 seconds
Diazepam	2.5–5 mg q2–4h	Undiluted	Inject 2–5 mg/minute
			Active metabolites contribute to activity
Diazoxide	50–150 mg q5–15 min	Undiluted	Inject over 30 seconds
			Maximum 150 mg/dose
Digoxin			
Digitalizing dose	0.25 mg q4–6h up to 1 mg	Undiluted	Inject over 3–5 minutes
Maintenance dose	0.125–0.25 mg q24h		Drug interactions: amiodarone, cyclosporine, quinidine, verapamil (8)
			Therapeutic levels: 0.5–2.0 ng/ml
Diltiazem			
Bolus dose	0.25–0.35 mg/kg	Undiluted	Inject over 2 minutes
Infusion dose	5–15 mg/hour	125 mg in D5W 100 ml	Continuous infusion (final concentration = 1 mg/ml)
Diphenhydramine	25–100 mg IV q2–4h	Undiluted	Inject over 3–5 minutes
			Competitive histamine antagonist, doses > 1000 mg/24h may be required in some instances

5.1 ▸ Intravenous Medication Administration Guidelines *(continued)*

Drug	Usual IV Dose Range*	Standard Dilution	Infusion Times / Comments / Drug Interactions
Dobutamine	2.5–20 μg/kg/minute	500 mg in D5W 250 ml	Continuous infusion
Dopamine			
Renal dose	< 5 μg/kg/minute	400 mg in D5W 250 ml	Continuous infusion
Inotrope	5–10 μg/kg/minute	400 mg in D5W 250 ml	Continuous infusion
Pressor	> 10 μg/kg/minute	400 mg in D5W 250 ml	Continuous infusion
Doxacurium			
Intubating dose	0.025–0.08 mg/kg	Undiluted	Inject over 5–10 seconds
Maintenance dose	0.005–0.01 mg/kg	Undiluted	Inject over 5–10 seconds
Infusion dose	0.25 μg/kg/minute	25 mg in D5W 50 ml	Continuous infusion Dose based on lean body weight Drug interactions: aminoglycosides (3); anticonvulsants (5)
Doxycycline	100–200 mg q12–24h	D5W 250 ml	Infuse over 60 minutes
Droperidol	0.625–10 mg q1–4h	Undiluted	Inject over 3–5 minutes
Enalaprilat	1.25–5 mg q6h	Undiluted	Inject over 5 minutes Initial dose for patients on diuretics is 0.625 mg
Epinephrine	1–4 μg/minute	1 mg in D5W 250 ml	Continuous infusion
Erythromycin	0.5–1 g q6h	NS 250 ml	Infuse over 60 minutes Drug interactions: theophylline (4); cyclosporine (9)
Erythropoietin	12.5–525 U/kg 3 × per week	Undiluted	Inject over 3–5 minutes

Drug	Usual IV Dose Range*	Standard Dilution	Infusion Times / Comments / Drug Interactions
Esmolol			
Bolus dose	500 μg/kg	Undiluted	Inject over 60 seconds
Infusion dose	50–400 μg/kg/minute	5 g in D5W 500 ml	Continuous infusion
Ethacrynic acid	50 mg	D5W 50 ml	Inject over 3–5 minutes
	May repeat $\times$ 1		Maximum single dose 100 mg
Etidronate	7.5 mg/kg qd $\times$ 3 d	NS or D5W 500 ml	Infuse over at least 2 hours
Famotidine	20 mg q12h	D5W 100 ml	Infuse over 15–30 minutes
Fentanyl			
Bolus dose	25–75 μg q1–2h	Undiluted	Inject over 5–10 seconds
Infusion dose	50–100 μg/hr	Undiluted	Continuous infusion
Filgastrim	1–20 μg/kg $\times$ 2–4 weeks	D5W	Preferred route of administration is subcutaneous
Fluconazole	100–800 mg q24h	Premix solution 2 mg/ml	Maximum infusion rate 200 mg/hour (IV rate is 15–30 minutes)
Flumazenil			
Reversal of conscious sedation	0.2 mg initially, then 0.2 mg q 60 seconds to a total of 1 mg	Undiluted	Inject over 15 seconds Maximum dose of 3 mg in any 1-hour period
Benzodiazepine overdose	0.2 mg initially, then 0.3 mg $\times$ 1 dose, then 0.5 mg q30 seconds up to a total of 3 mg	Undiluted	Inject over 30 seconds Maximum dose of 3 mg in any 1-hour period
Continuous infusion	0.1–0.5 mg/h	5 mg in D5W 1000 ml	Continuous infusion

5.1 ▶ Intravenous Medication Administration Guidelines *(continued)*

Drug	Usual IV Dose Range*	Standard Dilution	Infusion Times/Comments/Drug Interactions
Foscarnet			
Induction dose	60 mg/kg q8h	Undiluted	Infuse over 1 hour
Maintenance dose	90–120 mg/kg q24h	Undiluted	Infuse over 2 hours
Furosemide			
Bolus dose	20–40 mg q1–2h	Undiluted	Maximum injection rate 40 mg/minute
Infusion dose	3–15 mg/hour	100 mg in NS 100 ml	Continuous infusion
Gallium nitrate	100–200 mg/m² qd × 5d	D5W 1000 ml	Infuse over 24 hours
Ganciclovir	2.5 mg/kg q12h	D5W 100 ml	Infuse over 1 hour
Gentamicin			
Loading dose	2–3 mg/kg	D5W 50 ml	Infuse over 30 minutes
Maintenance dose	1.5–2.5 mg/kg q8–24h	D5W 50 ml	Infuse over 30 minutes
Single daily dose	5–7 mg/kg q24h	D5W 50 ml	Infuse over 30 minutes
			Critically ill patients have an increased volume of distribution requiring increased doses
			Drug interactions: neuromuscular blocking agents
			Therapeutic levels:
			Peak: 4–10 mg/L
			Trough: <2 mg/L
			Single daily dose: trough level at 24 hours = 0 mg/L; peak levels unnecessary
Glycopyrrolate	5–15 µg/kg	Undiluted	Inject over 60 seconds
Granisetron	10 µg/kg	D5W 50 ml	Infuse over 15 minutes

Drug	Usual IV Dose Range*	Standard Dilution	Infusion Times/Comments/Drug Interactions
Haloperidol (lactate)			
Bolus dose	1–10 mg q2–4h	Undiluted	Inject over 3–5 minutes
Infusion dose	10 mg/h	100 mg in D5W 100 ml	Continuous infusion
			In urgent situations the dose may be doubled every 20–30 minutes until an effect is obtained
			Decanoate salt is only for IM administration
Heparin	10–25 U/kg/hour	25,000 units in D5W 500 ml	Drug interactions: nitroglycerin (11)
Hydralazine	5–20 mg q4–6h	Undiluted	Inject over 3–5 minutes; doses every 30 minutes may be required for eclampsia
Hydrochloric acid	mEq = (0.5×BW × (103-serum Cl))	100 mEq in SW 1000 ml	Maximum infusion rate = 0.2 mEq/kg/hour
Hydrocortisone	12.5–100 mg q6–12h	Undiluted	Inject over 60 seconds
Hydromorphone	1–4 mg q4–6h	Undiluted	Inject over 60 seconds
			Dilaudid-HP available as 10 mg/ml
Imepenem	0.5–1 g q6–8h	D5W 100 ml	Infuse over 30–60 minutes
Isoproterenol	1–10 µg/minute	2 mg in D5W 500 ml	Continuous infusion
Ketamine			
Bolus dose	1–4.5 mg/kg	Undiluted	Inject over 60 seconds
Infusion dose	5–45 µg/kg/minute	200 mg in D5W 500 ml	Continuous infusion

5.1 ▸ Intravenous Medication Administration Guidelines *(continued)*

Drug	Usual IV Dose Range*	Standard Dilution	Infusion Times / Comments / Drug Interactions
Labetalol			
Bolus dose	20 mg q15min	Undiluted	Inject over 2 minutes
Infusion dose	1–4 mg/minute	200 mg in D5W 160 ml	Continuous infusion
Levothyroxine	25–200 mg q24h	Undiluted	Inject over 5–10 seconds
			IV dose = 75% of PO dose
Lidocaine			
Bolus dose	1 mg/kg	Undiluted	Inject over 60 seconds
Infusion dose	1–4 mg/minute	2 g in D5W 500 ml	Continuous infusion
			Drug interactions: cimetidine (6)
			Therapeutic levels: 1.5–5.0 mg/L
Lorazepam			
Bolus dose	0.5–2 mg q1–4h	Dilute 1:1 with NS before administration	Inject 2 mg/minute
Infusion dose	0.06 mg/kg/hour	20 mg in D5W 250 ml	Monitor for lorazepam precipitate in solution
			Use in-line filter during continuous infusion to avoid infusing precipitate into patient

Drug	Usual IV Dose Range*	Standard Dilution	Infusion Times/Comments/Drug Interactions
Magnesium (elemental)			Magnesium 1 g = 8 mEq
Magnesium deficiency	25 mEq over 24 hours followed by 6 mEq over the next 12 hours	25 mEq in D5W 1000 ml	Continuous infusion
Acute myocardial infarction	15–45 mEq over 24–48 hours followed by 12.5 mEq/day for 3 days	25 mEq in D5W 1000 ml	Continuous infusion
Ventricular arrhythmias	16 mEq over 1 hour followed by 40 mEq over 6 hours	40 mEq in D5W 1000 ml	16 mEq (2 g) may be diluted in 100 ml D5W and infused over 1 hour
Mannitol			
Diuretic	12.5–100 g over 1–2 hours	Undiluted	Inject over 3–5 minutes
Cerebral edema	1.5–2 g/kg over 30–60 minutes	Undiluted	Inject over 3–5 minutes
Meperidine	25–100 mg q2–4h	Undiluted	Inject over 60 seconds Avoid in renal failure
Metaraminol			
Bolus dose	0.5–5 mg	Undiluted	Inject over 60 seconds
Continuous infusion	20–500 µg/min	100 mg in NS 500 ml	Continuous infusion
Methadone	5–20 mg qd	Undiluted	Inject over 3–5 minutes Accumulation with repetitive dosing
Methyldopate	0.25–1 g q6h	D5W 100 ml	Infuse over 30–60 minutes

5.1 ▶ Intravenous Medication Administration Guidelines *(continued)*

Drug	Usual IV Dose Range*	Standard Dilution	Infusion Times / Comments / Drug Interactions
Methylprednisolone	10–500 mg q6h	Undiluted	Inject over 60 seconds
Metoclopramide			
Small intestine intubation	10 mg × 1	Undiluted	Inject over 3–5 minutes
Antiemetic	2 mg/kg before chemo, then 2 mg/kg q2h × 2, then q3h × 3	D5W 50 ml	Infuse over 15–30 minutes
Metoprolol	5 mg q2min × 3	Undiluted	Inject over 3–5 minutes
Metronidazole	500 mg q6h	Premix solution 5 mg/ml	Infuse over 30 minutes
Mezlocillin	3 g q4h	D5W 100 ml	Infuse over 15–30 minutes
Midazolam			
Bolus dose	0.025–0.35 mg/kg q1–2h	Undiluted	Inject 0.5 mg/minute
Infusion dose	0.5–5 µg/kg/minute	50 mg in D5W 100 ml	Continuous infusion Unpredictable clearance in critically ill patients Drug interactions: cimetidine (6)
Milrinone			
Loading dose	50 µg/kg	1 mg/ml	Infuse over 10 minutes Available in 5-ml syringe
Maintenance dose	0.375–0.75 µg/kg/minute	50 mg in D5W 250 ml	Continuous infusion

Drug	Usual IV Dose Range*	Standard Dilution	Infusion Times / Comments / Drug Interactions
Mivacurium			
Intubating dose	0.25 mg/kg	Undiluted	Inject over 60 seconds
Maintenance dose	0.1 mg/kg	Undiluted	Inject over 60 seconds
Infusion dose	9–10 μg/kg/minute	50 mg in D5W 100 ml	Continuous infusion
			Drug interactions: aminoglycosides (3); anticonvulsants (5)
Morphine			
Bolus dose	2–10 mg	Undiluted	Inject over 60 seconds
Infusion dose	2–5 mg/h	100 mg in D5W 100 ml	Continuous infusion
Nafcillin	0.5–2 g q4–6h	D5W 100 ml	Infuse over 30–60 minutes
Naloxone			
Bolus dose	0.4–2 mg	Undiluted	Inject over 60 seconds
	Max 10 mg		
Infusion dose	3–5 μg/kg/h	2 mg in D5W 250 ml	Continuous infusion
Neostigmine	25–75 μg/kg	Undiluted	Inject over 60 seconds
Nitroglycerin	10–200 μg/minute	50 mg in D5W 250 ml	Continuous infusion
			Drug interactions: heparin (11)
Nitroprusside	0.5–10 μg/kg/minute	50 mg in D5W 250 ml	Continuous infusion
			Maintain thiocyanate $<$ 10 mg/dl
Norepinephrine	4–10 μg/minute	4 mg in D5W 250 ml	Continuous infusion
Ofloxacin	200–400 mg q12h	D5W 100 ml	Infuse over 60 minutes

5.1 ▸ Intravenous Medication Administration Guidelines *(continued)*

Drug	Usual IV Dose Range*	Standard Dilution	Infusion Times / Comments / Drug Interactions
Ondansetron			
Chemotherapy-induced nausea and vomiting	32 mg 30 minutes before chemotherapy	D5W 50 ml	Infuse over 15–30 minutes
Postoperative nausea and vomiting	4 mg × 1 dose	Undiluted	Inject over 2–5 minutes
Oxacillin	0.5–2 g q4–6h	D5W 100 ml	Infuse over 30 minutes
Pamidronate	60–90 mg × 1 dose	D5W 1000 ml	Infuse over 24 hours
Pancuronium			
Intubating dose	0.06–0.1 mg/kg	Undiluted	Inject over 60 seconds
Maintenance dose	0.01–0.015 mg/kg	Undiluted	Inject over 60 seconds
Infusion dose	1 μg/kg/minute	50 mg in D5W 250 ml	Continuous infusion Metabolite contributes to activity Drug interactions: aminoglycosides (3); anticonvulsants (5)
Penicillin G	8–24 MU divided q4h	D5W 100 ml	Infuse over 15–30 minutes
Pentamidine	4 mg/kg q24h	D5W 50 ml	Infuse over 60 minutes
Pentobarbital			
Bolus dose	20 mg/kg	NS 100 ml	Infuse over 2 hours
Infusion dose	1 mg/kg/hour initially, then 0.5–3.5 mg/kg/hour	NS 250 ml 2g in NS 250 ml	Continuous infusion Therapeutic levels: 20–50 mg/L

Drug	Usual IV Dose Range*	Standard Dilution	Infusion Times/Comments/Drug Interactions
Phenobarbital Status epilepticus	20 mg/kg	Undiluted	Inject over 3–5 minutes Therapeutic levels: 15–40 mg/L

Phentolamine
  Bolus dose
  Continuous
    infusion
	2.5–10 mg prn
	1–5 mg/minute
		Undiluted
		50 mg in D5W 100 ml
			Inject over 3–5 minutes
			Continuous infusion

Phenylephrine	20–30 µg/minute	15 mg in D5W 250 ml	Continuous infusion; 0.5 mg over 20–30 seconds

Phenytoin
 	
  Status epilepticus
	15 mg/kg	Undiluted	Maximum infusion rate: 25 to 50 mg/minute
			Drug interactions: cimetidine (6); neuromuscular blocking
			  agents (5)
			Therapeutic levels: 10–20 mg/L

Phosphate
  (potassium)
	0.08–0.24 mmol/kg	Function of K$^+$
		  concentration
			Infuse over 6–8h
			1 mmol of PO$_4$ = P 31 mg
			Solution should be made no more concentrated than 0.4
			  mEq/ml of K$^+$

Piperacillin	2–4 g q4–6h	D5W 100 ml	Infuse over 15–30 minutes

Piperacillin/
  tazobactam
	3.375g IV q6h	D5W 100 ml	Infuse over 30 minutes
			Each 2.25-g vial contains 2 g piperacillin and 0.25 g
			  tazobactam

Plicamycin	15–25 µg/kg qd × 3–4 d	NS 1000 ml	Infuse over 4 to 6 hours

5.1 ▶ Intravenous Medication Administration Guidelines *(continued)*

Drug	Usual IV Dose Range*	Standard Dilution	Infusion Times/Comments/Drug Interactions
Potassium chloride	5–40 mEq/hour	40 mEq in 1000 ml (NS, D5W, etc)	Cardiac monitoring should be used with infusion rates > 20 mEq/hour
Prednisolone	4–60 mg q24h	Undiluted	Inject over 60 seconds
Procainamide			
Loading dose	15 mg/kg	D5W 50 ml	Maximum infusion rate 25–50 mg/minute
Infusion dose	1–4 mg/minute	2g in D5W 500 ml	Continuous infusion Therapeutic levels: Procainamide: 4–10 mg/L NAPA: 10–20 mg/L
Propofol			
Bolus dose	0.25–0.5 mg/kg	Undiluted	Infuse over 1–2 minutes
Infusion dose	5–50 μg/kg/minute	Undiluted	Continuous infusion
Propranolol			
Bolus dose	0.5–1 mg q5–15 min	Undiluted	Infuse over 60 seconds
Infusion dose	1–4 mg/hour	50 mg in D5W 500 ml	Continuous infusion
Protamine	<30 minutes: 1–1.5 mg/100 U; 30–60 minutes: 0.5–0.75 mg/100 U; > 120 minutes: 0.25–0.375 mg/100 U	50 mg in SW 5 ml	Inject over 3–5 minutes; do not exceed 50 mg in 10 minutes
Pyridostigmine	100–300 μg/kg	Undiluted	Use to reverse long-acting neuromuscular blocking agents Inject over 60 seconds

Drug	Usual IV Dose Range*	Standard Dilution	Infusion Times/Comments/Drug Interactions
Quinidine gluconate	600 mg initially, then 400 mg q2h, maintenance 200–300 mg q6h	800 mg in D5W 50 ml	Infusion rate 1 mg/minute; use cardiac monitor Therapeutic levels: 1.5–5 mg/L
Ranitidine			
IVPB	50 mg q6–8h	D5W 50 ml	Infuse over 15–30 minutes IVP dose should be injected over at least 5 minutes
Infusion dose	6.25 mg/hour	150 mg in D5W 150 ml	Continuous infusion
Rocuronium			
Intubating dose	0.45–1.2 mg/kg	Undiluted	Inject over 60 seconds
Maintenance dose	0.075–0.15 mg/kg	Undiluted	Inject over 60 seconds
Infusion dose	10–14 μg/kg/minute	50 mg in D5W 100 ml	Continuous infusion
Streptokinase			
Acute myocardial infarction	1.5 MU	D5W 45 ml	Infuse over 30 minutes
Deep venous thrombosis, pulmonary embolism	250,000 U over 30 minutes, then 100,000 U/hour over 24–72 hours	D5W 90 ml	Continuous infusion
Succinylcholine	0.6–2 mg/kg	Undiluted	Infuse over 60 seconds
t-PA	100 mg	100 mg in D5W 100 ml	Infuse 60 mg/hour during first hour, then 20 mg/hour for 2 hours
Thiamine	100 mg qd × 3	D5W 50 ml	Infuse over 15–30 minutes

5.1 ► Intravenous Medication Administration Guidelines *(continued)*

Drug	Usual IV Dose Range*	Standard Dilution	Infusion Times / Comments / Drug Interactions
Thiopental	3–4 mg/kg	Undiluted	Inject over 3–5 minutes
Ticarcillin	3g q3–6h	D5W 100 ml	Infuse over 15–30 minutes
Ticarcillin/clavulanate	3.1 g q4–6h	D5W 100 ml	Infuse over 15–30 minutes
Tobramycin			
Loading dose	2–3 mg/kg	D5W 50 ml	Infuse over 30 minutes
Maintenance dose	1.5–2.5 mg/kg q8–24h	D5W 50 ml	Infuse over 30 minutes
			Critically ill patients have an increased volume of distribution requiring increased doses
			Drug interactions: neuromuscular blocking agents (3)
			Therapeutic levels:
			Peak: 4–10 mg/L
			Trough: <2 mg/L
Torsemide	5–20 mg qd	Undiluted	Inject over 60 seconds
Trimethaphan	0.3–5 mg/minute	500 mg in D5W 500 ml	Continuous infusion
Trimethaprim-sulfamethoxazole			
Common infections	4–5 mg/kg q12h	TMP 16 mg-SMX 80 mg per D5W 25 ml	Infuse over 60 minutes
PCP	5 mg/kg q6h	TMP 16 mg-SMX 80 mg per D5W 25 ml	Infuse over 60 minutes
			Therapeutic levels: 100–150 mg/L

Drug	Usual IV Dose Range*	Standard Dilution	Infusion Times/Comments/Drug Interactions

Urokinase
  Pulmonary
    embolism
	4,400 U/kg over 10 minutes, then
	  4,400 U/h over 12 hours
		D5W 195 ml	Continuous infusion

Vancomycin	1 g q12h	D5W 250 ml	Infuse over at least 1 hour to avoid "red-man" syndrome
			Therapeutic levels:
			  Peak: 20–40 mg/L
			  Trough: <10 mg/L

Vasopressin	0.2–0.4 U/minute	100 units in D5W 250 ml	Maximum infusion rate 0.9 U/minute

Vecuronium
  Intubating dose
  Maintenance dose
  Infusion dose
	0.1–0.28 mg/kg
	0.01–0.015 mg/kg
	1 μg/kg/minute
		Undiluted
		Undiluted
		20 mg in D5W 100 ml
			Inject over 60 seconds
			Inject over 60 seconds
			Continuous infusion
			Metabolite contributes to activity
			Drug interactions: aminoglycosides (3); anticonvulsants (5)

Verapamil Bolus dose	0.075–0.15 mg/kg	Undiluted	Inject over 1–2 minutes Continuous infusion Drug interactions: digoxin (8)

5.2 ► Neuromuscular Blocking Agents

Agent	Dose	Onset/Duration	Comments
Depolarizing Agents			
Succinylcholine	Intubating dose: 1–2 mg/kg	Onset: 1 minute Duration: 10 minutes	Prolonged paralysis in pseudocholinesterase deficiencies Contraindications: Family history of malignant hyperthermia, neuromuscular disease, hyperkalemia, open eye injury, major tissue injury (burns, trauma, crush), increased intracranial pressure Side effects: bradycardia (especially in children), tachycardia, increased serum potassium concentration
Nondepolarizing Agents *Short-acting*			
Mivacurium	Intubating dose: 0.25 mg/kg	Onset: 5 minutes Duration: 15–20 minutes	Metabolized by pseudocholinesterase Intubating dose: initial 0.15 mg/kg followed in 30 seconds by 0.1 mg/kg
	Maintenance dose: 0.1 mg/kg Continuous infusion: 9.0–10.0 μg/kg/minute	Duration: 15 minutes	

Agent	Dose	Onset/Duration	Comments
Intermediate-Acting			
Atracurium	Intubating dose: 0.5 mg/kg	Onset: 2 minutes Duration: 30–40 minutes	Histamine release with bolus doses >0.6 mg/kg and may precipitate asthma or hypotension
	Maintenance dose: 0.08–0.10 mg/kg	Duration: 15–25 minutes	Elimination independent of renal or hepatic function Metabolized in the plasma by Hofmann elimination and ester hydrolysis
	Continuous infusion: 5–9 μg/kg/minute		Duration not prolonged by renal or liver failure Used when succinylcholine is contraindicated or not preferred
Rocuronium	Intubating dose: 0.45–1.2 mg/kg	Onset: 0.7–1.3 minutes Duration: 22–67 minutes	Not associated with histamine release Used when succinylcholine is contraindicated or not preferred
	Maintenance dose: 0.075–0.15 mg/kg	Duration 12–17 minutes	Metabolized by liver; duration not significantly prolonged by renal failure, but prolonged in patients with liver disease
	Continuous infusion: 10–14 μg/kg/minute		No adverse cardiovascular effects
Vecuronium	Intubating dose: 0.1–0.15 mg/kg	Onset: 2 minutes Duration: 30–40 minutes	Not associated with histamine release Bile is the main route of elimination
	Maintenance dose: 0.01–0.15 mg/kg	Duration 15–25 minutes	Metabolized by liver; minimal reliance on renal function, although active metabolite accumulates in renal failure
	Continuous infusion: 1 μg/kg/minute		Used when succinylcholine is contraindicated or not preferred No adverse cardiovascular effects

5.2 ► Neuromuscular Blocking Agents *(continued)*

Agent	Dose	Onset/Duration	Comments
Long-Acting			
Doxacurium	Intubating dose: 0.025–0.8 mg/kg Maintenance dose: 0.005–0.01 mg/kg Continuous infusion 0.25 µg/kg/minute (not generally recommended)	Onset: 4–5 minutes Duration: 55–160 minutes Duration 35–45 minutes	No adverse cardiovascular effects Predominantly renally eliminated; significant accumulation in renal failure
Pancuronium	Intubating dose: 0.06–0.1 mg/kg Maintenance dose: 0.01–0.015 mg/kg Continuous infusion: 1 µg/kg/minute (not generally recommended)	Onset: 2–3 minutes Duration 60–100 minutes Duration 25–60 minutes	Tachycardia (vagolytic effect) Metabolized by liver; minimal reliance on renal function, although active metabolite accumulates in renal failure

5.3 ▶ Vasoactive Agents

| Agent and Dose | Receptor Specificity | | | | | | Pharmacologic Effects | | | |
	α	β₁	β₂	DM	SM	VD	VC	INT	CHT	Comments
Inotropes										
Dobutamine										Useful for acute management of low cardiac output states; in chronic CHF intermittent infusions palliate symptoms but do not prolong survival
2–10 µg/kg/minute	1+	3+	2+	—	—	1+	1+	3+	1+	
>10–20 µg/kg/minute	2+	4+	3+	—	—	2+	1+	4+	2+	
Isoproterenol										Used primarily for temporizing treatment of life-threatening bradycardia
2–10 µg/kg/minute	—	4+	3+	—	—	3+	—	4+	4+	

α_1: α_1-adrenergic; β_1: β_1-adrenergic; β_2: β_2-adrenergic; DM: dopaminergic; SM: smooth muscle; VD: vasodilator; VC: vasoconstrictor; INT: inotropic; CHT: chronotropic.
Vasoconstrictors usually are given by central vein and should be used only in conjunction with adequate volume repletion. All can precipitate myocardial ischemia. All except phenylephrine can cause tachyarrhythmias.
Modified from: Gonzalez ER, Meyers DG: Assessment and management of cardiogenic shock. In Oronato JC (ed.): Clinics in emergency medicine: Cardiovascular emergencies. New York: Churchill Livingstone, 1986, p. 125, with permission.

5.3 ▸ Vasoactive Agents *(continued)*

Agent and Dose	Receptor Specificity			Pharmacologic Effects						Comments
	α	β₁	β₂	DM	SM	VD	VC	INT	CHT	
Amrinone 　Loading dose 　　0.75 mg/kg 　Maintenance dose: 　　5–15 µg/kg/minute	—	—	—	—	2+	2+	—	3+	3+	Useful for acute management of low cardiac output states; can be combined with dobutamine Associated with the development of thrombocytopenia
Milrinone 　Loading dose: 50 µg/kg 　　over 10 minutes 　Maintenance dose: 　　0.375–0.75 µg/kg/minute	—	—	—	—	2+	2+	—	3+	3+	Useful for acute management of low cardiac output states; can be combined with dobutamine
Mixed										
Dopamine 　2–5 µg/kg/minute 　5–10 µg/kg/minute 　10–20 µg/kg/minute	— — 3+	3+ 4+ 4+	— 2+ 1+	4+ 4+ —	— — —	— — —	— — 3+	2+ 4+ 3+	1+ 2+ 3+	Doses above 20–30 µg/kg/minute usually produce no added response; 2 µg/kg/minute may protect kidneys when giving other vasopressors
Epinephrine 　0.01–0.05 µg/kg/minute 　>0.05 µg/kg/minute	1+ 4+	4+ 3+	2+ 1+	— —	— —	1+ —	1+ 3+	4+ 3+	2+ 3+	Mixed vasoconstrictor/inotrope; stronger inotrope than norepinephrine; does not constrict coronary or cerebral vessels; give as needed to maintain BP

Agent and Dose	Receptor Specificity			Pharmacologic Effects						
	α	β_1	β_2	DM	SM	VD	VC	INT	CHT	*Comments*
Vasopressors										
Norepinephrine 2–20 μg/minute, titrate to effect	4+	2+	—	—	—	—	4+	1+	2+	Mixed vasoconstrictor/inotrope; useful when dopamine inadequate; give as needed to maintain BP (usually ≤20 μg/minute)
Phenylephrine Start at 30 μg/minute IV and titrate	4+	—	—	—	—	—	4+	—	—	Pure vasoconstrictor without direct cardiac effect; may cause reflex bradycardia; useful when other pressors cause tachyarrhythmias; give as much as needed to maintain BP
Metaraminol 0.5–5 mg slow IV bolus, titrate to effect	2+ − 3+	0	1+	0	—	0	3+	1+	1+	Predominant vasoconstrictor with mild inotropic effect; especially useful for shock associated with spinal anesthesia or CNS lesions
Vasodilators										
Nitroglycerin 20–100 μg/minute	—	—	—	—	4+	4+ A < V	—	—	1+	Tachyphylaxis, headache
Nitroprusside 0.5–10 μg/kg/minute	—	—	—	—	4+	4+ A = V	—	—	1+	Monitor thiocyanate levels if infusion duration >48 hours; maintain thiocyanate level <10 mg/dl

5.4 ► Antiarrhythmic Agents

Agents	Indications	Dosage	Comments
Class IA			
Procainamide	Ventricular ectopy; conversion of atrial fibrillation and atrial flutter; WPW	Loading dose: (IV) 15 mg/kg at 25–50 mg/minute, (PO) 1g Maintenance dose: (IV) 2–5 mg/minute; (PO): 500 mg q3h or SR 500–1500 mg q6h	N-acetyl procainamide is active metabolite; lupus-like syndrome; rash; agranulocytosis; QT prolongation Therapeutic range: PA 4–10 mg/L, NAPA 10–20 mg/L
Quinidine	Ventricular ectopy; conversion of atrial fibrillation and atrial flutter; WPW	Quinidine sulfate: 200–300 mg PO q6h Quinidine gluconate: 324–648 mg PO q8h	Diarrhea, nausea, headache, dizziness; hypersensitivity reactions including thrombocytopenia; hemolysis; fever; hepatitis; rash; QT prolongation; increased digoxin level Dosage adjustment should be made when switching from one salt to another: Quinidine sulfate (83% quinidine), gluconate (62% quinidine), polygalacturonate (60% quinidine) Therapeutic range: 2.5–5 mg/L
Disopyramide	Ventricular ectopy; conversion of atrial fibrillation and atrial flutter; WPW	100–300 mg PO q6h; SR: 100–300 mg PO q12h	Anticholinergic effects; negative inotropy; QT prolongation Therapeutic range: 2–4 mg/L

Abbreviations: MAT, multifocal atrial tachycardia; SR: Sustained release; SVT, supraventricular tachycardia; WPW, Wolff-Parkinson-White.

Agents	Indications	Dosage	Comments
Class IB			
Lidocaine	Malignant ventricular ectopy; WPW	1.5 mg/kg IV over 2 minutes, then 1–4 mg/minute	No benefit in atrial arrhythmias Seizures; paresthesias; delirium; levels increased by cimetidine; minimal hemodynamic effects Therapeutic range: 1.5–5 mg/L
Mexiletine	Malignant ventricular ectopy	150–300 mg PO q6–8h with food	No benefit in atrial arrhythmias Less effective than IA and IC agents Nausea; tremor; dizziness; delirium; levels increased by cimetidine Therapeutic range: 0.5–2 mg/L
Tocainide	Malignant ventricular ectopy	200–600 mg PO q8h with food	No benefit in atrial arrhythmias Less effective than IA and IC agents Nausea; tremor; dizziness; delirium; agranulocytosis; pneumonitis; minimal hemodynamic effects Therapeutic range: 4–10 mg/L

5.4 ▶ Antiarrhythmic Agents *(continued)*

Agents	Indications	Dosage	Comments
Class IC			
Flecainide	Life-threatening ventricular arrhythmias refractory to other agents Prevention of symptomatic, disabling, paroxysmal supraventricular arrhythmias, including atrial fibrillation or flutter and WPW in patients without structural heart disease	100–200 mg PO q12h	Proarrhythmic effects; moderate negative inotropy; dizziness; conduction abnormalities Therapeutic range: 0.2–1 mg/L
Propafenone	Life-threatening ventricular arrhythmias refractory to other agents SVT, WPW, and paroxysmal atrial fibrillation or flutter in patients without structural heart disease	150–300 mg PO q8h	Proarrhythmic effects; negative inotropy; dizziness; nausea; conduction abnormalities
Class IB/IC (hybrid electrophysiologic effects)			
Moricizine	Life-threatening ventricular arrhythmias refractory to other agents	100–300 mg PO q8h	Proarrhythmic effects; dizziness; nausea; headache
Class II (beta-blocking agents)			
Propranolol	Slowing ventricular rate in atrial fibrillation, atrial flutter, and SVT; suppression of PVCs	Up to 0.5–1 mg IV, then 1–4 mg/hour (or 10–100 mg PO q6h)	Not cardioselective; hypotension; bronchospasm; negative inotropy

Agents	Indications	Dosage	Comments
Esmolol	Slowing ventricular rate in atrial fibrillation, atrial flutter, SVT, and MAT	Loading dose: 500 μg/kg over 1 minute Maintenance dose: 50 μg/kg/minute; rebolus and increase q5min by 50 μg/kg/minute to maximum of 400 μg/kg/minute	Cardioselective at low doses; hypotension; negative inotropy; very short half-life
Metoprolol	Slowing ventricular rate in atrial fibrillation, atrial flutter, SVT, and MAT	Initial IV dose: 5 mg q5min up to 15 mg, then 25–100 mg PO q8–12h	Cardioselective at low doses; hypotension; negative inotropy
Class III Amiodarone	Life-threatening ventricular arrhythmias, supraventricular arrhythmias, including WPW refractory to other agents	800–1600 mg PO qd for 1–3 weeks, then 600–800 mg PO qd for 4 weeks, then 100–400 mg PO qd	Half-life >50 days; pulmonary fibrosis; corneal microdeposits: hypo/hyper-thyroidism; bluish skin; hepatitis; photosensitivity; conduction abnormalities; mild negative inotropy; increased effect of coumadin; increased digoxin level Therapeutic range: 1–2.5 mg/L
Bretylium	Refractory ventricular tachycardia and ventricular fibrillation	5–10 mg/kg IV boluses q10min up to 30 mg/kg, then 0.5–2 mg/minute	Initial hypertension, then postural hypotension; nausea and vomiting; parotitis; catecholamine sensitivity
Sotalol	Life-threatening ventricular arrhythmias	80–160 mg PO q12h; may increase up to 160 mg PO q8h	Beta blocker with Class III properties; proarrhythmic effects; QT prolongation

5.4 ▶ Antiarrhythmic Agents *(continued)*

Agents	Indications	Dosage	Comments
Class IV (calcium channel antagonists)			
Verapamil	Conversion of SVT; slowing ventricular rate in atrial fibrillation, atrial flutter, and MAT	IV bolus: 5–10 mg over 2–3 minutes (repeat in 30 minutes prn), continuous infusion: 2.5–5 µg/kg/minute PO: 40–160 mg PO q8h	Hypotension; negative inotropy; conduction disturbances; increased digoxin level; generally contraindicated in WPW
Diltiazem	Conversion of SVT; slowing ventricular rate in atrial fibrillation, atrial flutter, and MAT	IV bolus: 0.25 mg/kg over 2 minutes (repeat in 15 minutes prn with 0.35 mg/kg IV); Maintenance infusion: 5–15 mg/hour PO: 30–90 mg PO q6h	Hypotension; less negative inotropy than verapamil; conduction disturbances; rare hepatic injury; generally contraindicated in WPW
Miscellaneous Agents			
Adenosine	Conversion of SVT, including WPW	6 mg rapid IV bolus; if ineffective, 12 mg rapid IV bolus 2 minutes later; follow bolus with fast flush; use smaller doses if giving through central venous line	Flushing; dyspnea; nodal blocking effect increased by dipyridamole and decreased by theophylline and caffeine; very short half-life (≈ 10 seconds)

Agents	Indications	Dosage	Comments
Atropine	Initial therapy for symptomatic bradycardia	0.5 mg IV bolus; repeat q5 min prn to total of 2 mg IV	May induce tachycardia and ischemia
Digitalis	Slowing AV conduction in atrial fibrillation and atrial flutter	Loading dose: 0.5 mg IV, then 0.25 mg IV q4–6h up to 1 mg; Maintenance dose: 0.125–0.375 mg PO/IV qd	Heart block; arrhythmias; nausea; yellow vision; numerous drug interactions, generally contraindicated in WPW Therapeutic range: 0.5–2.0 ng/ml

5.5 ▶ Therapeutic Drug Monitoring

Drug	Usual Therapeutic Range	Usual Sampling Time
Antibiotics		
Amikacin	Peak: 20–40 mg/L Trough: <10 mg/L Single daily dose: 0 mg/L at 24 h	Peak: 30–60 minutes after a 30-minute infusion Trough: just before next dose Single daily dose: trough level just before next dose
Chloramphenicol	Peak: 10–25 mg/L Trough: 5–10 mg/L	Peak: 30–90 minutes after a 30-minute infusion Trough: just before the next dose
Flucytosine	Peak: 50–100 mg/L Trough: <25 mg/L	Peak: 1–2 hours after an oral dose Trough: just before next dose
Gentamicin	Peak: 4–10 mg/L Trough: <2 mg/L Single daily dose: 0 mg/L at 24 h	Peak: 30–60 minutes after a 30-minute infusion Trough: just before next dose Single daily dose: trough level just before next dose
Tobramycin	Peak: 4–10 mg/L Trough: <2 mg/L	Peak: 30–60 minutes after a 30-minute infusion Trough: just before next dose
Netilmicin	Peak: 4–10 mg/L Trough: <2 mg/L Single daily dose: 0 mg/L at 24 h	Peak: 30–60 minutes after a 30-minute infusion Trough: just before next dose Single daily dose: trough level just before next dose
Vancomycin	Peak: 20–40 mg/L Trough: <10 mg/L	Peak: 1 hour after end of a 1-hour infusion Trough: just before next dose
Sulfonamides (sulfamethoxazole, sulfadiazine, cotrimoxazole)	Peak: 100–150 mg/L	Peak: 2 hours after 1-hour infusion Trough: not applicable

Drug	Usual Therapeutic Range	Usual Sampling Time
Antiarrhythmics		
Amiodarone	0.5–2 mg/L	Trough: just before next dose
Digoxin	0.5–2 µg/ml	Peak: 8–12 hours after administered dose
		Trough: just before next dose
Disopyramide	2–4 mg/L	Trough: just before next dose
Flecainide	0.2–1.0 mg/L	Trough: just before next dose
Lidocaine	1.5–5 mg/L	Anytime during a continuous infusion
Mexiletine	0.5–2 mg/L	Trough: just before next dose
Procainamide/NAPA	Procainamide: 4–10 mg/L	IV: immediately after IV loading dose, anytime during continuous infusion
	NAPA: 10–20 mg/L	PO: trough: just before next dose
Quinidine	2.5–5 mg/L	Trough: just before next dose
Tocainide	4–10 mg/L	Trough: just before next dose
Anticonvulsants		
Carbamazepine	4–12 mg/L	Trough: just before next dose
Pentobarbital	20–50 µg/ml	IV: immediately after IV loading dose, anytime during continuous infusion
Phenobarbital	15–40 mg/L	Trough: just before next dose
Phenytoin	10–20 mg/L	IV: 2–4 hours after dose
		Trough: PO/IV: just before next dose
		Free phenytoin level: 1–2 mg/L

5.5 ▶ Therapeutic Drug Monitoring *(continued)*

Drug	Usual Therapeutic Range	Usual Sampling Time
Valproic acid	50–100 mg/L	Trough: just before next dose
Bronchodilators Theophylline	10–20 mg/L	IV: prior to IV bolus dose, 30 minutes after end of bolus dose, anytime during continuous infusion PO: peak: 2 hours after rapid-release product, 4 hours after sustained-release product Trough: Just before next dose
Miscellaneous Cyclosporine	50–150 ng/ml (whole blood, HPLC)	Trough: IV, PO: just before next dose

5.6 ► Tips for Calculating Intravenous Medication Infusion Rates

Information required to calculate intravenous infusion rates to deliver specific medication doses:
1. Dose to be infused (e.g., mg/kg/minute, mg/minute, mg/hour)
2. Concentration of intravenous solution (e.g., dopamine 400 mg in D5W 250 ml = 1.6 mg/ml; nitroglycerin 50 mg in D5W 250 ml = 200 μg/ml)
3. Patient's weight

A. Calculate the intravenous infusion rate in milliliters per hour for a 70-kg patient requiring dobutamine 5 μg/kg/minute using a dobutamine admixture of 500 mg in D5W 250 ml.
1. Dose to be infused: 5 μg/kg/minute
2. Dobutamine concentration: 500 mg/250 ml = 2 mg/ml or 2000 μg/ml
3. Patient weight: 70 kg
Calculation: 5 μg/kg/minute $\times$ 70 kg = 350 μg/minute
350 μg/minute $\times$ 60 minutes/hour = 21,000 μg/hour
21,000 μg/hour $\div$ 2000 μg/ml = 10.5 ml/hour
Answer: Setting the infusion pump at 10.5 ml/hour will deliver dobutamine at a dose of 5 μg/kg/minute.

B. Calculate the intravenous infusion rate in milliliters per hour for a 70-kg patient requiring nitroglycerin 50 μg/minute using a nitroglycerin admixture of 50 mg in D5W 250 ml.
1. Dose to be infused: 50 μg/minute
2. Nitroglycerin concentration: 50 mg/250 ml = 0.2 mg/ml or 200 μg/ml
3. Patient weight: 70 kg
Calculation: 50 μg/minute $\times$ 60 minutes/hour = 3000 μg/hour
3000 μg/hour $\div$ 200 μg/ml = 15 ml/hour
Answer: Setting the infusion pump at 15 ml/hour will deliver nitroglycerin at a dose of 50 μg/minute.

5.6 ▶ Tips for Calculating Intravenous Medication Infusion Rates *(continued)*

C. Calculate the intravenous loading dose and infusion rate in milliliters per hour for a 70-kg patient requiring aminophylline 0.6 mg/kg/hour using an aminophylline admixture of 1 g in D5W 500 ml. The loading dose should be diluted in D5W 100 ml and infused over 30 minutes.

  1. Desired dose: Loading dose: 6 mg/kg
     Maintenance infusion: 0.6 mg/kg/hour
  2. Aminophylline concentration:
     Aminophylline vial: 500 mg/20 ml = 25 mg/ml
     Aminophylline infusion: 1 g/500 ml = 2 mg/ml
  3. Patient weight: 70 kg

Calculation:
Loading dose: 6 mg/kg × 70 kg = 420 mg
420 mg ÷ 25 mg/ml = 16.8 ml
Infusion rate: Aminophylline 16.8 ml + D5W 100 ml = 116.8 ml
116.8 ml ÷ 0.5/hours = 233.6 ml/hour
Answer: Setting the infusion pump at 234 ml/hour will infuse the aminophylline loading dose over 1/2 hour
Maintenance dose: 0.6 mg/kg/hour × 70 kg = 42 mg/hour
42 mg/hour ÷ 2 mg/ml = 21 ml/hour
Answer: Setting the infusion pump at 21 ml/hour will deliver the aminophylline maintenance dose at 42 mg/hour, or 0.6 mg/kg/hour.

Miscellaneous

6.1 ► Healing Rituals for Relaxation, Music Therapy, Imagery, and Touch

Separation Phase
Before the Session

- Turn the radio and television off. To avoid interruptions, place a sign on the door stating that a session is in progress. (If other family members or significant others are around, invite them to join in and experience the intervention being taught to the patient.)
- Prepare the room to ensure as much comfort and quietness as possible.
- Have the patient tend to basic comfort needs, such as urinating, before the session begins.
- Ask the patient to sit, recline, or lie down, depending on preference and/or the situation.
- Have a light blanket available in case the patient should feel cool.
- Become calm and centered. Let your body-mind release any tension and tightness.
- Select a relaxation, imagery, music, or touch exercise (or combine these interventions) for the session.
- Ask the patient to notice baseline feelings/emotions before the session begins.

Beginning the Session

- Discuss the purpose of the session, reinforcing the intent of developing a positive expectation of what is to occur. This explanation helps individuals to focus and organize inner experiences towards calmness, inner harmony, and healing.

- Instruct the patient to focus on the present moment in order to facilitate the best relaxation, imagery, music, or touch experience.

- Encourage spontaneous images to emerge from the inner self without analyzing them. Should participants begin to analyze the images, instruct them to let the images just float on, and to release any logical process of resolving conflicts, establishing goals, and so forth. These steps will come, but not in a logical manner.

- Ask the patient to concentrate fully on the guided relaxation, imagery, music, and touch suggestions and instructions. Different images will emerge. If any image appears that is uncomfortable or that the patient is not ready to explore, provide instruction to let go of these images and flow with the next image that appears.

- Encourage the use of positive imagery that can evoke healing and healthy expectations.

- As you begin guiding the patient in a relaxation, imagery, music therapy, or touch experience, begin the experience with "You can let your eyes close to be fully awake or you can find a spot in front of you to focus on to begin to explore this experience of inner calmness. Allow the images to emerge from this relaxed state."

Transition Phase
During the Session

- Ask the patient to follow the suggestions that you give (or that are given on the tape that he or she will use for a session). Tell the patient to add his or her own suggestions that can allow more personal images to emerge. (If relaxation and different imagery states have been previously experienced, the individual will find it easier to clear the mind of distracting thoughts than if the individual is a beginner.)

- Inform the participant that with relaxation a decreased tension in the face, chest, torso, and legs will be experienced. The changes can be subtle or dramatic. Respirations become deeper with more space between the breaths. Eyelids may flicker especially if the patient is a vivid imager. Legs and feet will also turn outward with increased relaxation.

- If the mind cannot be cleared, suggest that the patient focus on slow, rhythmic, abdominal breathing. If the mind continues to wander, focus once again on the breathing pattern. It is natural for the mind to wander, and when aware of this, return to the relaxation, imagery, music therapy, or touch experience.

- The length of a session is based on the patient's needs, body responses, and session outcomes. The sessions can be 20 minutes or as long as needed. During the day encourage patients to incorporate relaxation, imagery, music, and touch skills in mini-sessions (3 to 5 minutes).

Return Phase
Closing the Session

- Gradually bring the patient back into full alertness by counting back from 5 to 1.
- Encourage the participant to become immersed in the healing silence and relaxed state even if only for a few minutes. The immediate period following a session can be a time for personal insight. This opportunity may be lost if patients begin talking or move into daily activities too soon.
- Instruction may be given to finish the session by drawing some images or writing some thoughts that occurred during the session.
- Ask the patient to interpret the experience. Ask open-ended questions about the *subjective experience* of relaxation, imagery, music therapy, and touch for further meaning or more personal insight about the current situation or other important issues.
- Encourage monitoring of tension during the day to replace tension patterns with relaxation and positive imagery. This is the body-mind communication process to enhance healing and recovery.
- Encourage awareness of the constant self-talk, and focus on creating positive images that lead to healthy outcomes.
- Recommend using "constant instant practice." This is a reminder to take a moment to practice, thereby integrating the practice into daily life.
- Explore the importance of trusting intuition and images that come forth from inner awareness.
- Encourage *practice*. This is the key to developing the deep levels of insight that can be gained from these healing strategies and rituals. Each day establish a scheduled time to practice. Just as one takes medication on a schedule, a scheduled relaxation, imagery, touch, or music session increases personal skills.
- Alternate between short and long practice sessions.

6.2 ► Intracranial Pressure Waveforms

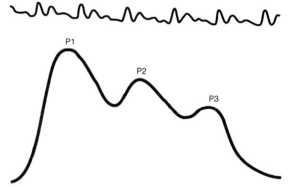

A. Normal ICP waveforms. P1 = percussion wave; P2 = tidal wave;
P3 = dicrotic wave.

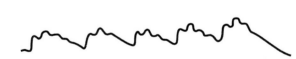

B. ICP waveform with poor compliance

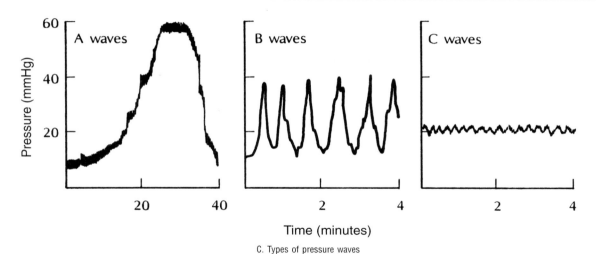

C. Types of pressure waves

6.3 ► Complications of Enteral Feeding

Complications	Cause	Therapeutic Interventions
GI Complications		
Diarrhea	Low-residue formula	Select fiber formula
	Rapid formula administration	Initiate feeding at low rate
		Temporarily reduce rate
	Bolus feeding using syringe force	Reduce rate of administration; select alternative method
	Hypoalbuminemia	Use elemental or peptide-based formula or total parenteral nutrition until absorptive capacity of gut is restored
	Microbial contamination	Use good handling and administration technique
	Disuse atrophy	Use enteral nutrition whenever possible
	Rapid GI transit time	Select fiber formula; slow transit time
	Prolonged antibiotic treatment or other drug therapy	Review medical profile and eliminate causative agent if possible; question benefit of lactobacillus
	Nutrient malabsorption	Select formula that restricts offending nutrients
Cramping, gas, abdominal distention	Rapid, intermittent administration of refrigerated formula	Administer formula by continuous method and at room temperature
	Bolus feeding using syringe force	Reduce rate of administration; select alternative method
Nausea and vomiting	Rapid formula administration, gastric distention	Initiate feedings at low rate and gradually advance to desired rate of administration; temporarily reduce rate
		Consider postpyloric feeding tube
Constipation	Inadequate fluid intake	Supplement fluids
	Insufficient bulk	Fiber
	Inactivity	Get out of bed

Complications	Cause	Therapeutic Interventions
Metabolic Complications		
Dehydration	Inadequate fluid intake or excessive losses	Supplement fluid intake; monitor I&O
Overhydration	Rapid refeeding, excessive fluid intake	Reduce rate of administration, especially in patients with severe malnutrition or major organ failure; monitor I&O
Hyperglycemia	Inadequate insulin production for the amount of formula given Stress	Initiate feedings at low rate; monitor glucose; use oral hyperglycemia agents or insulin if necessary; select low-carbohydrate diet
	Inadequate fluid intake or excessive losses	Assess fluid and electrolyte status; supplement with appropriate fluid; monitor I&O
Hypernatremia	Inadequate intake, fluid overload, SIADH, excessive GI fluid losses	Assess fluid and electrolyte status; if necessary restrict fluids; use diuretics; replace with fluids of similar composition
Hyponatremia	Delayed gastric emptying, gastroparesis	Postpyloric feeding; select isotonic or low-fat formula; check residuals; reduce infusion rate; use concentrated formulas
Aspiration pneumonia	Gastrointestinal reflux, diminished gag reflex	Use small-bore feeding tubes to minimize compromise of LES HOB > 45° Initially and regularly check tube placement

6.3 ▶ Complications of Enteral Feeding *(continued)*

Complications	Cause	Therapeutic Interventions
Mechanical Complications		
Feeding tube plugging	Administering crushed medications	Administer as many medications in sorbitol-free elixir form as possible
		If crushing medications, make sure medications are finely crushed and tube is adequately flushed before and after delivery
		Use laser-bore tube for medication administration
	Administering sorbitol-based elixirs	Use sorbitol-free elixirs when available
		Adequately flush feeding tube
	Infrequent flushing of tube	Flush tube every 3–4 hours with warm water
		Flush tube before and after use with warm water
		If tube plugs, attempt to flush gently with warm water

6.4 ► Transport Personnel and Equipment Requirements

Personnel

A minimum of two people should accompany the patient.

One of the accompanying personnel should be the critical care nurse assigned to the patient or a specifically trained critical care transfer nurse. This critical care nurse should have completed a competency-based orientation and should meet the described standards for critical care nurses.

Additional personnel may include a respiratory therapist, registered nurse, critical care technician, or physician. A respiratory therapist should accompany all patients requiring mechanical ventilation.

Equipment

The following minimal equipment should be available.
- Cardiac monitor/defibrillator.
- Airway management equipment and resuscitation bag of proper size and fit for the patient.
- Oxygen source of ample volume to support the patient's needs for the projected time out of the ICU, with an additional 30-minute reserve.
- Standard resuscitation drugs: epinephrine, lidocaine, atropine.
- Blood pressure cuff (sphygmomanometer) and stethoscope.
- Ample supply of the IV fluids and continuous drip medications (regulated by battery-operated infusion pumps) being administered to the patient.
- Additional medications to provide the patient's scheduled intermittent medication doses and to meet anticipated needs (e.g., sedation) with appropriate orders to allow their administration if a physician is not present.

(From: American Association of Critical-Care Nurses: Guidelines for the transfer of critically ill patients. Aliso Vieja, CA: AACN, 1993.)

6.4 ► Transport Personnel and Equipment Requirements *(continued)*

- For patients receiving mechanical support of ventilation, a device capable of delivering the same volume, pressure, and PEEP and an Fio_2 equal to or greater than that the patient is receiving in the ICU. For practical reasons, in adults an Fio_2 of 1.0 is most feasible during transfer because this eliminates the need for an air tank and air-oxygen blender. During neonatal transfer, Fio_2 should be precisely controlled.

- Resuscitation cart and suction equipment need not accompany each patient being transferred, but such equipment should be stationed in areas used by critically ill patients and be readily available (within 4 minutes) by a predetermined mechanism for emergencies that may occur en route.

6.5 ▶ Monitoring During Transfer

- If technologically possible, patients being transferred should receive the same physiological monitoring during transfer that they were receiving in the ICU.
- Minimally, all critically ill patients being transferred must have continuous monitoring of ECG and pulse oximetry and intermittent measurement and documentation of blood pressure, respiratory rate, and pulse rate.
- In addition, selected patients, based on clinical status, may benefit from monitoring by capnography; continuous measurement of blood pressure, PAP, and ICP; and intermittent measurement of CVP, Pao, and CO.
- Intubated patients receiving mechanical support of ventilation should have airway pressure monitored. If a transfer ventilator is used, it should have alarms to indicate disconnects or excessively high airway pressures.

From: American Association of Critical-Care Nurses: Guidelines for the transfer of critically ill patients. *Aliso Viejo, CA: AACN, 1993.*

6.6 ▶ Pretransfer Coordination and Communication

- Physician-to-physician and/or nurse-to-nurse communication regarding the patient's condition and treatment preceding and following the transfer should be documented in the medical record when the management of the patient will be assumed by a different team while the patient is away from the ICU.

- The area to which the patient is being transferred (X-ray, operating room, nuclear medicine, etc.) must confirm that it is ready to receive the patient and immediately begin the procedure or test for which the patient is being transferred.

- Ancillary services (e.g., security, respiratory therapy, escort) must be notified as to the timing of the transfer and the equipment and support needed.

- The responsible physician must be notified either to accompany the patient or to be aware that the patient is out of the ICU at this time and may have an acute event requiring the physician's response to provide emergency care in another area of the hospital.

- Documentation in the medical record must include the indication for transfer, the patient's status during transfer, and whether the patient is expected to return to the ICU.

From: American Association of Critical-Care Nurses: Guidelines for the transfer of critically ill patients. *Aliso Viejo, CA: AACN, 1993.*